Children's Written Language Difficulties

Children's Written Language Difficulties
Assessment and Management

Edited by
Margaret J. Snowling

First published 1985
by The NFER-Nelson Publishing Company Ltd.
Reprinted 1989, 1990, 1991

Reprinted 1993 and 1994
by Routledge
11 New Fetter Lane, London EC4P 4EE

© 1985 Margaret J. Snowling

Printed and bound in Great Britain by
Antony Rowe Ltd, Chippenham, Wiltshire

British Library Cataloguing in Publication Data
A catalogue record for this book is available from the British Library

ISBN 0-415-09872-6

Contents

List of Figures   vi
List of Tables   vii
List of Contributors   viii
Preface   ix
Introduction: 1
   Children with specific learning difficulties: the role of the speech
   therapist   Jean M. Cooper   3

Part 1:   The clinical picture   9

Chapter 1   What is dyslexia? A developmental language
           perspective   Harry Chasty   11
Chapter 2   Verbal deficits in dyslexia: a review   John Rack and
           Margaret Snowling   28
Chapter 3   The question of prevention   Peter Bryant   43

Part 2:   Procedures for the assessment and management of children
          with reading and spelling difficulties   57

Chapter 4   The assessment of some persisting language difficulties
           in the learning disabled   Hanna Klein   59
Chapter 5   The assessment of reading and spelling skills
           Margaret Snowling   80
Chapter 6   Segmentation, speech and spelling difficulties
           Joy Stackhouse   96

Part 3:   Approaches to the treatment of reading and spelling
          difficulties   117
Chapter 7   A structured phonetic/linguistic method for teaching
           dyslexics   Beve Hornsby   119
Chapter 8   Extending the written language skill of children with
           specific learning difficulties – supplementary teaching
           techniques   Nata Goulandris   134
Chapter 9   Guidelines for teachers, parents and learners   Jean
           Augur   147

Postscript: 171
   Some consistencies and contradictions: directions for future
   research   Margaret Snowling   173

References   175
Index   185

Figures

Chapter 1   Figure 1.1 In early language development   12
            Figure 1.2 Later language system (after age 5+)   13
            Figure 1.3 Illustration of anomalous chest of drawers   19
            Figure 1.4 'News' written by 7-year-old boy   21
            Figure 1.5 Spelling of a 7-year-old boy   22
            Figure 1.6 Figure relating student ability to level of
                        developing language structure   24

Chapter 2   Figure 2.1 Two-store model of memory (after Atkinson
                        and Shiffrin, 1968)   35
            Figure 2.2 Serial position curve   36

Chapter 4   Figure 4.1 Illustration of cards used for teaching tables
                        in a multisensory manner   76
            Figure 4.2 An extract from 'The Romans' by Joan Forman   77

Chapter 5   Figure 5.1 Information processing model of the reading
                        process   86
            Figure 5.2 Information processing model of the spelling
                        process   90
            Figure 5.3 Phonetic spelling from a teenage dyslexic   91
            Figure 5.4 Free writing from a 10-year-old who makes
                        nonphonetic spelling errors   91

Chapter 6   Figure 6.1 Two-route model of the reading process (after
                        Coltheart, 1980)   98
            Figure 6.2 Model of the spelling process (after Frith,
                        1980)   100

Chapter 7   Figure 7.1 Examples of 'Alpha to Omega' flashcards:
                        consonants   122
            Figure 7.2 Flashcards from 'Alpha to Omega': vowels   123
            Figure 7.3 Free writing from David, aged 6 years 7
                        months, Verbal I.Q. 123   128
            Figure 7.4 Spelling and free writing produced by Noel,
                        aged 8 years, Verbal I.Q. 107   129
            Figure 7.5 Spelling and free writing produced by
                        Christopher, aged 11 years 10 months   131

Figure 7.6 Free writing from Mary, aged 17 years,
Verbal I.Q. 125   133

Chapter 8   Figure 8.1 Examples of some useful mnemonics   139
Figure 8.2 Illustrations for spelling pattern 'ew'. Drawn
by a dyslexic child to help him learn the
spellings   140
Figure 8.3 Free writing from a 12-year-old girl   145

Chapter 9   Figure 9.1 A 12-year-old boy writing about those things
which he finds difficult   150
Figure 9.2 Examples of art work from a boy aged 11 and
a girl aged 8, both dyslexic   151
Figure 9.3 Page from a record book which documents a
child's reading progress   158
Figure 9.4 Alphabet friezes recommended for
reinforcement of letter names, sounds and
shapes   161
Figure 9.5 Example of helpful marking   163
Figure 9.6 Examples of unhelpful marking   164
Figure 9.7 Examples of a boy's writing attempts (1)
before tuition (2) a few months later (3) two
years later   169

Tables

Chapter 3   Table 3.1 Percentage of unexpectedly high and low
scorers on initial sound categorization tests
who became unexpectedly good and poor
readers (Neale)   48
Table 3.2 Percentage of unexpectedly high and low
scorers on initial sound categorization tests
who became unexpectedly good and poor
readers (Schonell)   48
Table 3.3 Percentage of unexpectedly high and low
scorers on initial sound categorization tests
who became unexpectedly good and poor
spellers (Schonell)   48

Chapter 4   Table 4.1 Naming errors made by Clifford, C.A. 9 years
8 mths   63
Table 4.2 Errors made by Linda, aged 11, on a picture-
naming task   70

Chapter 5   Table 5.1 Regression equation based on a primary
school population for ages 6–12 years (Yule *et
al*, 1982)   85
Table 5.2 Predicted Reading Ages (Neale Analysis of
Reading Ability: Accuracy score) and Spelling
Ages (Vernon test) in a primary school
population   85

Contributors

JEAN AUGUR is head of the Staines Remedial Education Centre, Knowle Green, Staines, Surrey.

PETER BRYANT is Watts Professor of Psychology, University of Oxford, Department of Experimental Psychology.

HARRY CHASTY is Director of Studies, The Dyslexia Institute, 133, Gresham Rd., Staines, Middlesex.

JEAN COOPER is Principal, National Hospitals College of Speech Sciences, 59, Portland Place, London W1.

NATA GOULANDRIS is a therapist at the Dyslexia Clinic, St. Bartholomews Hospital, London, and a research student at University College, London.

BEVE HORNSBY is a Speech Therapist and Psychologist who runs The City of London Dyslexia Charity Centre, 71, Wandsworth Common Westside, London SW18.

HANNA KLEIN is a speech and language therapist who specializes in the treatment of children and adolescents with specific learning difficulties in Surbiton, Surrey.

JOHN RACK is involved in research in the Department of Psychology, University College, London.

MARGARET SNOWLING is Professor of Psychology at the University of Newcastle upon Tyne.

JOY STACKHOUSE is Senior Lecturer in Speech Pathology, School of Speech Therapy, Department of Health Sciences, City of Birmingham Polytechnic, Birmingham.

Preface

The idea for this book came about as the result of a conference, *Speech Therapy and Specific Learning Difficulties: Present Trends*, convened by the British Dyslexia Association and held in conjunction with the National Hospitals College of Speech Therapists in October 1984.

The conference brought together speech therapists, teachers and psychologists, all keen to improve the methods they use for the assessment and management of children with specific learning difficulties/dyslexia. This is clearly an area of growing interest, especially amongst speech therapists in the United Kingdom. The focus was upon children whose problems with reading and spelling follow a history of (spoken) language difficulty – a group which speech therapists are particularly likely to encounter.

The chapters of the book have been developed from papers given at the conference, and additions have been made in response to delegates' comments during discussion. The authors are grateful to Daphne Hamilton-Fairley, Mary Manning-Thomas and Mary Nash-Wortham who shared their expertise on a discussion panel during the conference, and to Graham Cranmere, H.M.I. and Lord Halsbury, President, College of Speech Therapists, who chaired sessions.

Margaret J. Snowling

January, 1985

Introduction

Jean M. Cooper

Children with Specific Learning Difficulties: the Role of the Speech Therapist

Awareness of and commitment to the needs of individuals with various learning disabilities, particularly language-based learning difficulties, have increased greatly in the last decade and emphasized the importance of effective intervention from a variety of professional sources.

Those involved in the training of workers in this field certainly attempt to develop an individual who has an understanding of the handicap. Even more importantly, they develop a person who has both a clear perception of his own role in the intervention process and who has the ability to interact effectively with other disciplines. Developing this clear perception of one's role in the intervention process must not become confused with defending professional roles and responsibilities, as this can be detrimental to the children needing an integrated intervention programme and also to the specialists serving those children.

Before examining the role of speech therapy in the management of learning difficulties, it might be helpful to consider in general terms the concept of learning disability and the relationship of language to that disability.

'Learning disabilities' is a general term that refers to a diverse group of developmental and educational disorders. The National Advisory Committee on Handicapped Children, in the U.S.A., has used the following definition of the learning disabled child:

> Children with special learning disabilities exhibit a disorder in one or more of the basic psychological processes involved in understanding or in using spoken or written language. These may be manifest in disorders of listening, thinking, talking, reading, writing, spelling and arithmetic. They include conditions which have been referred to as perceptual handicaps, brain injury, minimal brain dysfunction, dyslexia, developmental aphasia etc. They do not include learning problems which are due primarily to visual, hearing or motor handicaps, to mental retardation or to environmental disadvantage.

This definition reflects the view that language is fundamental to academic learning.

Longitudinal research studies indicate that disorders of language comprise the majority of learning disabilities and this perhaps accounts for what might be termed a 'chicken and egg' situation. Which comes first? Are we talking about children with learning disability who demonstrate a language problem, or children with language disability who demonstrate a learning problem? It is interesting for example that the prevalence figures of language disorders in pre-school children appear to decline in the school aged population but that other learning disabilities begin to emerge at this stage. We could suggest that the early intervention work on oral language (both comprehension and production) with pre-school children accounts for this, but is this necessarily the true explanation? Perhaps instead the nature of the language problem changes and, whilst the child's oral language ability might have responded to intervention, the underlying problems that caused this processing difficulty might now be making it difficult to deal with other forms of language, namely reading and writing. Various studies indicate that children with early or oral language difficulties frequently maintain some form of communication problem even into early adulthood – i.e. a notion of continuum of failure.

The relationship between implicit and explicit language needs to be explored. Implicit language knowledge involves the abstraction and use of the linguistic rules for speaking and listening and explicit language knowledge involves the ability to examine these rules. It may be that the implicit language knowledge is enhanced, indeed increased by these early intervention strategies, but that problems persist with the high level language skills (sometimes referred to as metalinguistic skills) which involve explicit language knowledge.

The young child can be helped to apply rules to encode and decode meaning in sentences, to recognize and construct the syntax of sentences and to analyse and organize the spoken form of the utterance. This system of rules and strategies operates most efficiently without conscious awareness. However, learning to read and write requires the language-user's knowledge of phonology, syntax and semantics at a more conscious level. It seems therefore that two kinds of skill are required. Mattingley (1972) has called these a) 'primary linguistic activity', i.e. the ability to apply a set of internalized unconscious rules to the production and comprehension of sentences, and b) 'linguistic awareness', i.e. the ability to talk about language and analyse its components.

Our education system assumes that a child entering school has acquired an oral language system and therefore the design and formulation of the curriculum is based on this assumption. In recent years considerable attention has been paid to the content of the language used in the classroom and all of this research has emphasized the central role of language learning. Because language underlies the major portion of academic learning and is the primary means through which the curriculum is presented, the assessment of a child's skills in this area is crucial. Where learning difficulties are manifest a multidisciplinary team of professionals must be involved in the design and formation of the curricula, paying particular attention to the language interactions required for each specific learning task.

Although considerable information has been acquired about the nature of learning, about communication processes and about interferences in learning and communication, additional research is needed to meet the needs of individuals working in this field. In particular, what is needed is definitive research in the area of improved procedures to facilitate *early* identification. Prevention of learning difficulties is of course the ultimate aim, but this is extremely difficult to achieve. However, if we know that certain abilities are pre-requisites to the learning process, then we have some means of predicting likely problems. Better still, if we can improve these pre-requisite abilities, then we might have some means of preventing the problems.

Let us now return to the task of attempting to identify the contribution of speech therapy in the area of learning disabilities and of the learning process in general. Increased co-operation with teachers and psychologists has stimulated many speech therapists to look at their responsibilities, particularly in relation to reading and writing.

In 1972 the Quirk Report (the Committee appointed by the Secretary of State for Education and Science, for Social Services, for Scotland and for Wales in 1977) made the following recommendations:

> It was suggested to us in evidence that speech therapy could assist with a variety of learning problems, particularly difficulty in learning to read, even when no overt speech or language disorder was present. In particular, it was suggested that children suffering from specific reading difficulty (sometimes called 'Dyslexia') had often shown an earlier history of delayed or disordered language development.
>
> We have no wish to enter the present controversy about the nature, and indeed the existence of 'Dyslexia', nor into the question of the relevance of speech therapy to learning problems of this kind, though we expect the profession as a whole to maintain an interest in this field, and individuals perhaps to participate in research in it. There is little doubt, however, that the learning problem of a child suffering from word-sound difficulties associated with retarded development of language ability will be lessened by any treatment designed to accelerate the development of language. When a child who has been seen because of abnormal language development attends school for the first time, the speech therapist should, as a matter of routine, ensure that the teachers concerned are aware of the history of the language difficulty.
>
> We therefore recommend that speech therapists should ensure that teachers are informed of a history of late or impaired language development, to alert them to the possibility of future learning problems, but should not at present attempt to give further professional help unless an overt disorder of language is present.

It is now over a decade since this report was published and it is evident that the time has now come to re-examine carefully the speech therapist's role in relation to this field of disability. Certainly there is a strong nucleus of opinion which insists that speech therapists do involve themselves in the wider context of language disabilities, and there are many very experienced therapists working in this field today. Let us consider the contribution this profession might make in relation to language-based learning disabilities in terms of diagnosis, remediation and prevention.

One obvious rationale put forward to define the role of the speech therapist in remedying reading disabilities has been that the child with a reading problem may have a speech problem as well. In addition some experts claim that a reading disorder or other learning disability may originate in an underlying deficit of auditory skills and that specific auditory training is considered part of a speech therapist's skills.

These explanations, however, provide the speech therapists with only a limited role and it is hoped that the foregoing comments about learning in general and reading in particular and their relationship to oral language, together with the recent advances in speech sciences, indicate a rather wider scope of involvement.

The following extract from a paper by Rees (1974) sums up the contribution that speech therapists can make, not only in terms of practice but also in terms of planning and research:

> The speech pathologist has as his domain all aspects of speech and language, particularly the establishment of the internalized rules that constitute language competence, and the application of those rules to understanding and producing appropriate spoken utterances. The speech pathologist has the responsibility to assess language skills and identify the nature and extent of language deficits, as well as to make appropriate referrals and to design and carry out plans of intervention aimed at bringing the child up to his capacities in language skills. The speech pathologist's approach is based on the model of semantic, syntactic and phonological aspects of language. He has available to him a wide battery of test materials to assess the child's linguistic performance in all three areas and from which to make intelligent inferences about what the child knows about his language. The speech pathologist is armed with normative data about the maturational stages of linguistic skill in these areas, as well as teaching strategies for establishing new linguistic behaviours. The speech pathologist, in short, has the responsibility for developing in the child the linguistic prerequisites for reading that Mattingly (1972) termed "Primary Linguistic Activity".

Although the last word has not been said on either the theoretical or the clincal aspects of this issue, certainly the recent explosion of normative and clinical information about children's language has provided for language specialists a wealth of data and principled teaching methods.

It is also important, however, to recognize that the clinical/ educational management of reading and writing disorders is a specialized skill and requires explicit training. Therefore the speech therapists' involvement will of course depend on the value and extent of their training in this area. Current curricula of the various programmes leading to certification to practise as a speech therapist may need to give greater emphasis to this. Perhaps it is of even greater importance that continuing education courses of a multidisciplinary nature should more fully develop the competences required.

In summary, it must be emphasized that no one discipline has all the information necessary to provide all the service needed for the learning-disabled population, but in the best interests of this population, multidisciplinary management is advocated, and the speech therapist has a *vital* role in that management team.

Part 1

The Clinical Picture

Harry Chasty

1 What is Dyslexia? A Developmental Language Perspective

Terminology

Early approaches to understanding dyslexia stemmed from the work of medical researchers such as James Hinshelwood. From 1900 onwards he contributed a series of articles to the medical journals before publishing his book 'Congenital Word Blindness' in 1917. Hinshelwood believed that dyslexic children suffered from a congenital disorder associated with the left cerebral hemisphere of the brain which prevented the normal development of reading skill in children who were otherwise able and intelligent. It is from this early perspective that present understanding of this learning difficulty has developed. Some of the problems faced by practitioners currently working in the field arise from the fact that dyslexia was originally described by medicals, is now diagnosed by psychologists, while the provision of 'treatment' is in the hands of speech therapists and teachers.

Terminology can be very difficult. Hinshelwood's label 'Word Blindness' still found acceptance in 1963, when the Invalid Children's Aid Association opened the 'Word Blind Research Centre'. This unit was destined to have a marked effect upon the general acceptance of the disorder, and made a considerable contribution to the understanding of the psychological assessment and teaching of the dyslexic person. In the past twenty years, theory and practice have changed greatly and the label 'word blindness' is no longer acceptable because these children are not blind, and their visual acuity does not contribute to their reading difficulty. However, there is still much unnecessary acrimony over the alternative labels 'dyslexia' and 'specific learning difficulty'. Parents and voluntary organizations working in the field seem to prefer the term 'dyslexia', while the Department of Education and Science and local education authorities use 'specific learning difficulty' to refer to the problem.

This linguistic warfare is often conducted with a level of animosity which would not be out of place if it were described in 'Gulliver's Travels'! However, it is now generally accepted that children with this disorder are present in schools in considerable numbers, that the problems faced are recognizable, and that providing them with the teaching support they need is more important than arguing about what they should be called (or indeed whether they merit a descriptive label at all).

This more pragmatic attitude is reflected in the very practical views expressed in a recent report prepared by the British Psychological Society's Division of Educational and Child Psychologists. This report recommends, 'We must talk to those in other disciplines on the topic of specific learning difficulty, and be prepared to accept that they may wish to use the term 'dyslexia' even though we prefer SLD. We are keener to place the emphasis on the teaching programme than on the label used at this stage in our understanding of the processes involved'.

The purpose of this present chapter is to describe this complex concept of either 'dyslexia' or 'SLD' in detail so that the 'understanding of the processes involved' may be assisted, so leading to fuller recognition for dyslexics and a better teaching provision to meet their special educational needs.

Communication leads to Literacy

Babies are born helpless and totally dependent on others for all their needs, and this gives impetus to the development of an effective communication system between the child and those in his immediate environment. Even from birth the child has thoughts which may be expressed as feelings rather than words or pictures, but are nevertheless equally real and valid. 'I am hungry; I need to be fed.' 'I am lonely; I need someone to cuddle me.' 'I am uncomfortable; I need someone to change me.' So the child cries and a perceptive parent understands, and sees to his needs. Over a period of time the infant learns that his wants will be more effectively met if he uses his muscle system with some skill, to turn his 'ma . . .' into a more winsome and appealing 'ma ma'. This

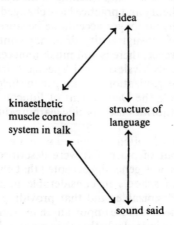

Figure 1.1 In early language development

leads to the development of a repertoire of sounds used each time to convey a particular idea for the child.

The child progresses through babbling, the use of organized sound patterns which approximate to words, words used holophrastically, telegraphic speech. His utterances gradually become more skilled, more diffuse and wide-ranging, and much better for expressing his thoughts with precision.

This system is shown diagrammatically in Figure 1.1. The child's ideas are expressed through his expanding language structure by means of muscle control as sounds in talk, and those in his immediate environment listen and can understand his thoughts.

Teacher relies greatly upon this system when the child comes to school. She can say, 'Johnny, sit down' and he knows that 'Johnny' means him and that 'sit down' means that he must keep his bottom on that chair until told otherwise. Teacher's sounds have been turned reasonably effectively into ideas in Johnny's head. Equally, he can use this system too. He can say, 'Please, I need a pencil.' Already he will have modified his language structure to include the required school jargon. Teacher, who wants him to get on with his picture quietly, can meet that expressed need.

Once this system has been established with certainty, teacher sets about expanding it in its present form. However, later she makes a significant addition, a new element which completely revolutionizes the system. She gradually builds onto the child's existing structure of language a recognition of the printed forms of words he knows, so leading into reading. Expressing ideas this way has many advantages. In particular, it allows communication over time and distance. The

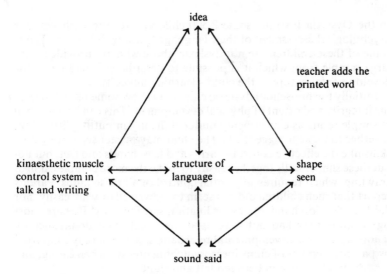

Figure 1.2 Later language system (after age 5 +).

shape '*Jane*', written today, can be shown to Mummy tonight or posted to Grandpa in Australia.

Figure 1.2 shows how the initial 'talk' system has been extended to provide a structure for reading. If teacher is doing her job well she will not only teach that *Jane* says 'J–a–n–e', linking shape with sound; she will also point out that *Jane* means that long-haired girl on page 9 of Ladybird Book 1A. She should make all the Janes in the class stand up so that the child links the shape of the word with its meaning. At a slightly later stage in the child's career she must also link that shape *Jane* with the moving pattern which must be written on paper to represent the idea permanently for others.

Over a period of time teacher will use either 'Look and Say' or 'phonics' to build links between the shape of the word seen and its sound. Both these methods are inappropriate for children who do not remember shapes or sounds well, and for them it will be necessary to link instantly and reinforce the bonds between shape, sound, writing pattern and meaning, teaching in what has been described as a multisensory way. However, to think of dyslexia only in terms of reading failure is grossly to over-simplify the complexity of the language development process. Dyslexia represents failure in a developmental communication system. It is in the pre-school stage that the major components of the literacy failure of the dyslexic child can first be identified.

Pre-school Aspects of the Problem

Physical organization

In the Dyslexia Institute some 2,500 children are seen each year for psychological assessment of their language learning difficulties. While some of these children are not dyslexic, those who are provide a very large sample from which it is possible to describe in broad terms the developmental nature of the child's learning difficulty.

Initially the pre-school dyslexic child may show some retardation in the integrity and extent of physical development. This can be described in simple terms as experiencing undue difficulty in putting little skills together to make a bigger skill. The child may master separately little skills like the effective control of arms and legs, hands and feet, but not put these simple skills together easily to make the more complex skill of crawling, which requires sequential control of all these limbs. Parents report that such children did not seem to crawl well or walk easily, nor did they develop hand–eye co-ordination satisfactorily. Perhaps most significantly they had not developed the usual hand dominance by school age. These developmental retardations are generally supported by parental reports of clumsiness, switching utensils when eating, and fundamental confusion between left and right.

It should not be forgotten that there is an essential 'physical' element in language. Muscles must be controlled in sequence with considerable skill to convey meaning in talk. A different set of muscles has to be moved effectively to express ideas in print when writing 'News'. The intensity of fine manipulative skill required over a prolonged period in an 'A' level written examination should not be underestimated.

The definition of language given by the Open University as 'the application of a public signal system to a sensori-motor capacity' is noted. The dyslexic child may well have the background language experience to familiarize him with the public signal standing for the idea he wishes to express, but not have the basic sensori-motor capacity required to produce the signal consistently. The poorly co-ordinated child who does not sequence and organize little skills effectively to make big skills is at risk in this area of language development.

Psychologists are well aware of the importance of this ability to build simple skills together to make larger skills and refer to it as 'schema formation'. Schema building is the foundation of more sophisticated abstract thinking because it permits the mature student to operate the cluster of skills making up the schema by a single action or thought. This leads to much greater efficiency in thinking and significantly higher speeds of information processing.

One of the major schemata or strategies which the child must develop is control over his preferred hand to make marks with a writing implement. This consists of seven separate actions which are learned independently by the child, and then sequenced into the correct order to complete the activity successfully. Eyes must be focussed on the pencil; the preferred arm stretched out the required distance; a hand lowered close to the pencil; finger and thumb must be opposed to grasp; the hand must pull the pencil in; it must be manipulated into the action mode; and finally a mark can be made on paper.

Initially each of these actions must be thought about and controlled separately, careful sequencing being vital in the successful completion of the action. As the child's hand skill develops, he eventually welds these seven separate physical actions into a unit controlled by a single thought – "make a mark" – and the pencil is manipulated to produce the required response.

Adults can carry out this activity automatically while thinking of other things, and it is this high level of schema control which makes such complex activities as essay writing possible. I can write my signature in the appropriate place on a cheque, producing a complicated motor pattern which is recognizable every time to my bank, while my main focus of attention is on some complex problem such as the fact that continued spending at this rate will have me broke long before pay day comes around again!

In tracing the thread which runs through the pre-school dyslexic child's development, and which later flaws his higher literacy skill development, it is necessary to look carefully for the child's initial difficulty in building fine motor, memory and language schemata, and the frequency of breakdown of these schemata under pressure.

Short-term memory

The concept of the schema, and the role it plays in idea-building, is also relevant in memory. Indeed, the word 'schema' was first used by Head and later by Bartlett in their classical description of the act of remembering. In 'Remembering', Bartlett defines the schema as 'an active organization of past reactions or past experiences which must always be supposed to be operating in any well-adapted organic response'. It is the reproduction of these organized models of past experience, or schemata, which constitutes the act of remembering. Memory is very much a question of model-building. This cannot be forgotten in making sense of the cognitive and language difficulties shown by the dyslexic child.

THE SHORT-TERM MEMORY SHELF IN PROBLEM-SOLVING

The importance of short-term memory in problem-solving can be appreciated from an analysis of how you, as an adult, might solve the sort of problem you must face frequently every day. Your gas fire is not working. The Gas Board promised to send a plumber to fix it last Thursday. You waited all day, but he did not come. It is cold in your flat and you need that fire. How will you solve the problem?

Initially you must talk to someone at the Gas Board. To do that, you must look up the appropriate six-figure string of digits in a telephone directory, and retain those digits for the limited period necessary for you to dial the number successfully. Can you hold that six-figure string of digits on your short-term memory shelf while carrying out that task, or do you have to adopt a somewhat slower and less efficient strategy and write the number sequence down on a sheet of paper so that you can look at it while you dial? Your shelf width will determine the speed at which you get through to the Gas Board.

As soon as the number rings and the telephonist answers, 'Gas Board', that set of digits is not just irrelevant, it is in your way. So you immediately discard the set of digits and put on your shelf a set of questions or strategies you intend to follow. (1) Why did the plumber not come? (2) When will he come? (3) What will he do? (4) How much will it cost? (5) Will it be a proper job?

Some of the answers are important and get transferred to long-term memory for storage and use at a later stage, (2), (3) and (4). Questions (1) and (5) are much less important and these answers will probably be discarded. You can see that your short-term memory shelf width determines the size of the information processing package you can handle, and the speed and efficiency of your handling, but does *not* determine how cleverly you can deal with the particular question. Once the information is on that shelf you may think about it at an extremely high level. Getting it on the shelf and keeping it there while it is thought about is another matter. This helps us understand why young dyslexic children can carry out some skills at a high level but will, on other skills where short-term memory is important, fail most unexpectedly.

THE USE OF SHORT-TERM MEMORY IN LANGUAGE LEARNING

Testing carried out with younger children from dyslexic families, i.e. those where older siblings have been assessed and found to be dyslexic, and where the parents themselves admit to having suffered similar language-learning difficulties, suggest that these children have early perceptual problems in both visual and auditory modalities.

In perception the sound or shape to be recognized must be retrieved from long-term memory and matched with the incoming stimulus on the short-term shelf. If the child has an inefficient auditory or visual short-term memory, he may fail to make the accurate match which allows him to interpret sound or shapes with the consistency necessary for efficient speaking or reading. The dyslexic child may have an auditory or visual perceptual difficulty which requires skilled teaching even in the pre-school years.

Despite sounds being accurately recognized, in the English language these simple sounds do not convey the meaning. They are patterned or organized into longer, more complex, groupings to provide meaning. The same three sounds are used in 'pat', 'tap' and 'apt', but the meaning of each combination is very different. A sense of order and organization in language is essential to get the meaning.

In listening to and extracting the sense of spoken language, the pre-school child must store a large chunk of speech so that it can be analysed in a sequential way. In the early stages, meaning is related to word order in the sentence. The regular subject–verb–object form enables the young child to make sense of who did what to whom, as in 'The dog bites the man'. Commenting on this development, Slobin (1971) points out that a similar subject–verb–object structure is observable in the early sentences of Russian children, although the adult Russian word order is generally subject–object–verb. In all child language, the organization used to produce and make sense of speech is not a direct reflection of the system used by the adults encountered in the child's background, but is determined by the child's own analysing and organizing experience. So analysis and organization shape the structure of the child's speech and determine the efficiency with which he both extracts sense from what is said to him and conveys his ideas in words. The child must use short-term memory to facilitate the analysis which leads to appreciation of the meaning triggers (or 'phrase markers') which indicate that a transformation has occurred, as in the sentence, 'The dog was bitten by the man'. The child is therefore engaged in applying his own particular grammatical rules to analysis of language material held in short-term memory every time he listens, speaks or reads. Equally he is also engaged in revising and modifying his existing language structure in the light of the continuous experience he undergoes.

Paula Menyuk (1963, 1969) studied the spontaneous speech of children aged three to six years. A group of these children has been described as using 'infantile' language. Her analysis indicated that these children were using deviant rather than infantile language. On a sentence imitation task she showed that her normal children were affected by sentence complexity but *not* by sentence length. Indeed, normal three-year-old children were able to reproduce sentences up to nine words long. In contrast, the sentence imitations made by her deviant group were determined by length of sentence. There was a strong relationship (+ 0.53) between sentence length and the deviant language group's inability to make the sentence. Menyuk noted that these children showed clear evidence of impaired auditory short-term memory. She concluded that in children who are unable to keep three morphemes in memory, linguistic analysis of incoming data is severely impaired. These children with impaired auditory short-term memory will produce utterances which are not only impoverished and limited, but possibly based upon different hypotheses and rules to those generated by 'normal' children.

In simple terms, the pre-school child with auditory short-term memory difficulty builds a different and less efficient model of language which impairs later language usage.

There is further evidence in the literature to support the view that the specific learning difficulties child who has a short-term memory deficit has an impaired language model. Wiig, Semel and Crouse (1973) reported significant differences between poor and normal readers aged nine on Berko's test of morphological usage. The errors made by the poor readers were considered to be idiosyncratic, and less predictable than those of normals. Wiig, Semel and Crouse conclude that syntactic deficiencies are significant precursors of reading failure and are a possible cause rather than a result of reading difficulty. They recommend that remediation of such deficiencies be undertaken prior to formal reading instruction in the infant class.

Vogel (1974) compared normal and dyslexic children on nine measures of spoken language, and found that the dyslexics were inferior on seven of the nine measures. Vogel's results supports the findings of Wiig *et al*, (op.cit), that poor appreciation of the structure of language and deficient reading skill are significantly related and have a common base.

Repeated observation of the speech of many dyslexic children shows that they may face difficulties and retardations in three areas. They may have very early difficulty with the production of particular sounds. Later on, they may experience some difficulty with the consistent sequencing of sounds into the required order in longer, multisyllabic words. A word such as 'susceptible' may be produced as 'suspectible', or 'car park' appears as 'par cark'.

More significantly, some dyslexic children experience serious difficulty in expressing ideas coherently in words in an efficient sentence. When shown a picture with something missing, the dyslexic child may recognize the missing item instantly (see Figure 1.3). His visual problem-solving may be fast and precise. However, when asked to express the idea in words the efficiency with which he carries out that task may be low. Instead of replying that 'The right-hand knob of the second drawer is missing', the dyslexic child may reply, 'It's that thing there, that you would hold on to if you wanted to open it'. Young dyslexics tend to use language to express meaning implicitly rather than explicitly. These children also experience some difficulty in defining words exactly. They may be familiar with the ideas, and know what the word means, but cannot express the idea effectively in spoken language for others. This inability to express ideas coherently is a serious restriction to the child's development when he enters the talk-orientated background of infant and junior school classrooms. But the problem has ramifications which go beyond simple communication. If the child cannot say it, he will not read it, write it or spell it. As Menyuk, Wiig and Vogel have suggested, there is a structural language base to reading difficulty.

We have seen that in the pre-school stage these children may show physical organizational problems, perceptual difficulties, auditory and visual short-term memory difficulties and display different use of spoken language skills. These traits are testable and recognizable before the child goes to school and before he learns to read. The narrow cognitive problems described will have effects at home and in school, and the child will present a rather enigmatic picture, doing some things rather well and others incompetently. However, it is necessary now to focus our attention on his development in school.

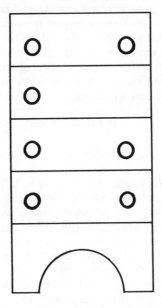

Figure1.3 Anomalous chest of drawers

The Dyslexic Child in School

The dyslexic child enters the 'buzzing, booming confusion' of the infant school classroom, bringing with him his generally unrecognized learning difficulties. Many teachers are still inadequately trained to deal with information processing problems in these children. The structured play and pre-reading training usually provided is not sufficient to overcome the organizational weakness which the child experiences. When the rest of the group moves on to pre-reading training, the dyslexic child is still in teacher's judgement 'not ready'. He may be held back to enable 'maturation' to bring about the desired competence, but the application of direct teaching to his physical, memory, perceptual and talk deficiencies is rare.

Eventually he will be asked to look at, recognize and recall shapes and apply a sound to a particular shape. As the child does not have the basic information processing tools to tackle this task, his failure in reading is to be expected. 'Look and Say' and 'phonic analysis' are inadequate methods to teach children experiencing the difficulties already described. The child's reading progress is slow and uncertain and his attitude to the printed word becomes increasingly hostile. At this stage in the child's development he can be described as having a reading difficulty, but this label will so grossly distort teacher's perspective by diverting attention from what is essentially a developmental language disorder, that its application can be positively harmful.

Reading is about turning symbols in sequence into sounds and extracting the meaning. Teacher is also working to develop other related skills. The child is being encouraged to express *his* ideas in sequence in symbols written on paper. It sounds complicated but is generally referred to by teacher and child as 'News'. The dyslexic child has difficulty in locating where he should start on the page, has problems in controlling the required letter shapes, has great difficulty in turning his bright ideas into verbal form, and experiences severe problems in translating the shape/sound idea of the word into the movement pattern for letters. For any idea he will have great difficulty in linking its shape with both the sound and the movement pattern for writing.

Figure 1.4 shows the News written by a 7-year-old boy of superior intellectual ability who is being educated in a good local education authority school. He can be relied upon to knock over the jar as he reaches for the Black Beauty pencil, trip over his friend's schoolbag as he returns to his desk, lick the pencil before writing and put a black streak from the corner of his mouth to his ear. When looking at his work one can almost hear his cry of aggravation as he abandons the 'I' on the right hand side of the top line and begins again on the left hand side of the page. He shows poor control of the pencil, making many letter shapes the wrong way round, and is very uncertain about spacing on the page. Letter size fluctuates greatly and quite unaccountably he leaves an immense gap in the middle of the page.

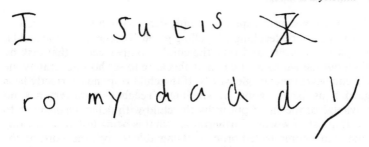

to the Sh r n

and   p u t   t he

e g o n the boo t

Figure 1.4 The 'News' written by a 7-year-old boy of superior intellectual ability. Note the abandoned attempt to start on the right side of the page, the difficulty in spacing, poor control of the pencil in letter production, and variation in the size of the letters. His ideas are good but are inadequately expressed. He writes: 'I sometimes row my daddy to the shore and put the engine on the boat.'

Increasingly as school loads the pressure on written work, the dyslexic child may show spelling difficulties.

Figure 1.5 shows the spelling of the same 7-year-old boy. His difficulties and confusions are clearly evident. He is subject to many letter reversals and confuses 'u' and 'a'. His directional problems are acute. In spelling 'Dad' he is aware that he is an important person who merits a capital letter, but places it at the end of the word. He wrote the dictated word 'good' as 'buog', writing right-handed from left to right. When questioned about the sound at the beginning of the word, he asked, 'Where is begin? What does "begin" mean?' It is impossible to spell or indeed read and write accurately until one is certain of where begin is and what it means.

Generally in schools, spelling is only dealt with in the most cursory fashion, with little teaching of spelling given. Teacher gives the child a list of words to learn and tests the child's competence at that task by calling out the words next day and checking to see how accurately the child can write these single words. If the child responds correctly he is regarded as being 'good at spelling'. Teacher, however, has no knowledge of the effort put in by the child with defective memory to learn that list of words. Furthermore, what is being tested is only one sub-skill in a complicated process. Being able to spell the word on the next day does not mean that the child will be able to spell it a week later, and spelling it the next day when required to write it quickly while thinking about other complicated ideas is not guaranteed. What is important is not the correct short-term production of the simple spelling sub-skill, but the effective use of that sub-skill as a sequential item in a long and complicated action schema such as story or essay writing.

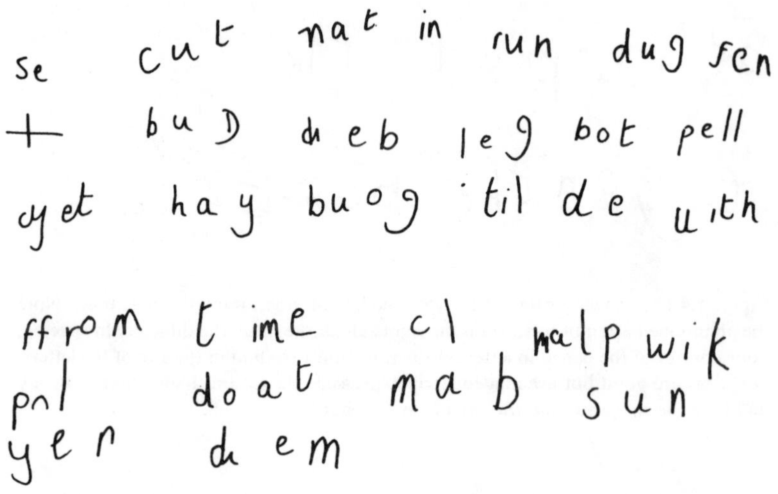

Figure 1.5 The spelling of a 7-year-old boy of superior ability. The words he printed are:

see	cut	mat	in	ran	bag	ten
hat	dad	bed	leg	dot	pen	
yet	hay	good	till	be	with	
from	time	call	help	week		
pie	boat	mind	sooner			
year	dream					

Note the printing of 'good', which is completely reversed.

Some 70 per cent of dyslexics experience difficulties with number language. The boy whose News and spelling has been shown certainly did. He could count with fingers or counters in practical terms. His trend to reversals resulted in his producing figures such as ⤴ and ⤸ , and confusions were evident between 2 and 5, 6 and 9. His directional problems caused difficulty in working out where to start. Sequencing right to left, down to up, up to down as well as left to right was too much for him. His short-term memory weakness affected his storage and retrieval of information from the question. Number facts, components and tables were not recalled with the efficiency necessary for accurate computation on paper.

So, in the classroom, reading, writing, studying, comprehension exercises, note-writing, essay writing, using tables, number facts, drawing maps, handling chemical formulae, learning foreign languages – all may be affected. The major problem to be faced in describing the classroom effects of dyslexia is that dyslexic children do not all show a standard group of weaknesses. Even close relatives such as twins or brothers may be impaired in different problem-solving areas. Too much attention should not be given to this variation between students which arises from interaction between the degree of dyslexia experienced, the student's ability, and personality factors such as motivation, interests and work habits. These varied symptoms are the outward secondary effects of inefficiency in brain organization which leads to uncertain control over higher language schemata.

Dyslexia may therefore be defined as an organizing difficulty which is usually congenital, but occasionally acquired; which affects physical skill development in laterality, information processing in short-term memory and perception, and so causes significant interference in the development of language in the individual. By language we mean talk, reading, spelling, writing, number, and essay writing.

Central to this concept of dyslexia is the idea of a developmental language disorder. As the child grows, each successive bit of his learning takes account of and uses what has gone before to build more complex skills. Developing language becomes intertwined in this structure, reinforcing, shaping and extending the child's thinking.

The schema building which has gone into motor skill development makes possible fine control of the articulatory musculature, so facilitating talking. Similar development with the dominant hand accommodates writing. Talk is the necessary foundation of reading, and the links between shape and sound, kinaesthetic pattern and meaning established in reading lead to writing, spelling, comprehension, studying and essay writing. Attainment in the education system depends upon the integrity of this structure.

The difficulty observed in the dyslexic student as he builds this cognitive structure is attributable to the information processing problems previously described which may be either reduced or increased by the intelligence and application which a student brings to bear upon the particular learning situation he faces. Students of high

student ability

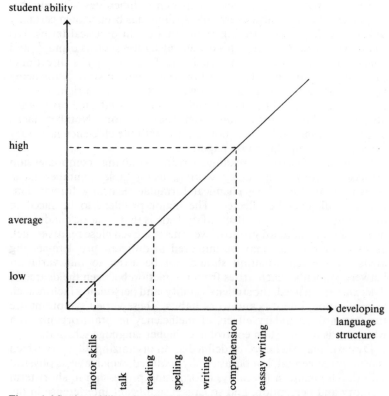

Figure 1.6 Student ability related to level of developing language structure

intellectual capability may have experienced slight uncertainty as they approached each new learning task, but because of their superior ability overcame the difficulty and added that skill or schema to their repertoire.

In looking at the special educational needs of dyslexic students in our education system it is necessary to take into account the kind of ability/degree of difficulty/language development relationship implied in Figure 1.6.

On the horizontal axis of the diagram developing language is represented, starting with motor skills and culminating in essay writing. On the vertical axis is presented the student's ability, ranging from low to high.

Low ability students will have difficulty starting at motor skills and experience problems at each successive stage. They will probably struggle greatly with reading, spelling and writing, and fail to build the detailed schemata necessary for comprehension and essay writing. The average ability dyslexic student will manage the motor skills and talk aspects of the continuum with slight delay, but will experience serious problems with reading and the stages which follow. The high ability student will manage the early stages of the continuum quite effectively and will only experience difficulty on the more complex language schemata such as comprehension, study skills, note writing and essay writing at the extreme right hand side of the development profile.

Adult dyslexics experiencing difficulty in the higher literacy skills are seen quite frequently at the Dyslexia Institute. Two cases particularly deserve mention.

The first young man was aged twenty-one and had achieved reasonable success in 'O' level examinations. However, he had taken 'A' level in Physics, Chemistry and Biology consistently for three years and had failed all three examinations each time. His tutors considered him to be an excellent practical scientist in every way. He had the information in his head, but seemed to be unable to produce it in the right sequence through his fingertips to satisfy his examiners.

Psychological testing showed that he was of superior intellectual ability, but had weakness in auditory and visual short-term memory, slight sequencing difficulty and signs of poor motor control skills. His reading aloud sounded quite skilled, but he had difficulty in answering searching questions about a text that he had just read aloud perfectly. Retention of meaning in comprehension was uncertain. Spelling was slightly suspect and speed of writing was rather slow. This young man reported that he was initially slow to learn to read, but by the age of nine he was as good as all the others in his class and his teacher certainly did not consider him to have a reading difficulty, even though he later found that he needed to read his scientific text books very carefully if he was to retain the sense. When questioned about his spelling skill he replied that he was usually regarded as an efficient speller, being able to score nine or ten out of ten most mornings on the spelling test. However, he pointed out that he found the Friday test, which took in the spellings learnt for the whole week, to be much more difficult and often did much less well on that. At the age of nine it certainly was not apparent that he had a learning difficulty, and he would have passed the screening tests applied by most local education authorities to spot children with specific learning difficulties.

In 'O' levels he had managed to get as much information as he could about the subject into his examination script and had been relatively successful. In 'A' levels, however, the standard required in the expression of ideas in writing is much higher and it is necessary to use information in a carefully sequenced and organized way to answer the precise question. This he could not do. Although the young man knew his information, he could not present it at the required level to satisfy his examiners, and his subsequent succession of failures was a very traumatic experience for him.

He was a bright, able dyslexic who had coped effectively with the early language schemata but failed to build an essay writing technique. He asked very searchingly, 'Whose job is it to give me the higher writing skills I need to prepare me for my scientific career?' He was well beyond compulsory school age and his education authority did not want to know about his difficulty. His problems were too specialized for the Adult Literacy Scheme and this is where the voluntary bodies working in the field of dyslexia fill a vital role by offering the highly specialized tuition which is not generally available through any other educational agency.

The man in the second case was aged thirty-five and had a relatively successful academic career, of which the only distinguishing factor was an inexplicable underachievement in the later stages. In his chosen profession he was a successful practitioner and was highly regarded by his colleagues and partners. In the final examination for membership of his professional body he unaccountably failed, and on the advice of his examiners came forward for psychological testing. He too was a very intelligent man, with competent reading, spelling and handwriting skills, but he had the short-term memory, sequencing and motor control difficulties usually seen in the cognitive background of the dyslexic person. He could produce very adequate reports when at leisure in his office, but under the intense strain of his professional examination, when his brain was preoccupied with handling extremely complex ideas at great speed, his spelling, writing and essay writing schemata fell apart and what he wrote did not do justice to his distinguished practical record.

These two cases show educational problems which are just as valid as those faced by the non-reading seven-year-old in the junior school or the slow reading, poor spelling, haphazard writing early teenager in the comprehensive school. The concept of dyslexia held by teachers and speech therapists should be sufficiently developed to provide for 'pre-school', 'in-school' and adult needs, and offer not just recognition but appropriate educational treatment.

The perspective on dyslexia presented here has been that of an ongoing organizing difficulty which has developmental language effects. These may be debilitating at successive stages or even the final stage of a person's educational career. The point in learning at which the difficulty first becomes obvious will be determined by the person's ability and the extent of his difficulty. The educational provision for these students should be individually determined yet related to the wide-ranging needs which have been described, opening rather than closing communication channels. The dyslexic student needs assessment, encouragement, skilled teaching and careful educational management, not placement in the younger, duller or slower learning group.

In his thinking course, Edward de Bono describes a father who, when confronted by the problem of his toddler son who insisted on tangling Granny's knitting, placed the playpen round Granny rather than round his son! Father realized that being placed in the playpen would be a restriction on the child's learning, but being placed in the playpen would present no such problem to Granny within her normal range of activities. Dyslexic students are often placed in a language playpen in an educational system which still regards knowledge as being that which a student can write down in neat sentences. It is to be hoped that, with the reappraisal brought about by the 1981 Education Act, schools and education authorities will take a similarly inspired approach to the education of the dyslexic children who fall within their area of responsibility.

John Rack and Margaret Snowling

2 Verbal Deficits in Dyslexia: a Review

In recent years, experimental psychologists have taken two different starting points for the investigation of developmental dyslexia. Perhaps the most popular has been to examine the perceptual and cognitive characteristics of diagnosed 'dyslexics' and to compare them with normal readers. The assumption underlying this approach is that any deficit uncovered and found to be *specific* to dyslexic individuals must account for the dyslexic condition. If this were true there would be important practical implications – early detection of dyslexia (before reading failure) would be possible, allowing for intervention and, at best, prevention of the difficulties.

Morrison and Manis (1983) point out a number of theoretical problems for this 'deficit' account of dyslexia. They identify questions of 'specificity and severity'. One question is, why should a process deficit primarily affect the task of reading, and how is it that dyslexic children can perform adequately in other tasks? A second problem is that of specifying the mechanisms by which a process deficit could influence the acquisition of literacy. A final problem is the question of direction of causality. For example, it is quite possible to argue that certain cognitive abilities develop as a consequence of the developing reading skills of the child, rather than to say that those cognitive skills dictate the course of reading development.

An alternative approach to the whole issue has been to investigate the reading and spelling processes characteristic of dyslexic individuals. It is usually assumed that identification of deficient strategies allows direct inference to be made about the underlying deficits which cause dyslexia. From a practical point of view, it is frequently argued that there are immediate treatment implications from such analysis. In fact, whether it is more beneficial to treat a deficient reading or spelling process, or alternatively, to promote a compensatory strategy which can circumvent the deficient one, remains open to question.

Both approaches to the study of dyslexia have generated an abundance of research. It is not the purpose of this chapter to review this extensive literature but rather to present converging evidence in support of the verbal deficit hypothesis of dyslexia (Vellutino, 1979). Before doing so, it is necessary to address some of the methodological issues which beset work in this area and about which there is not necessarily agreement.

Probably the most critical methodological question is that of control groups. Should dyslexic individuals be compared with normal readers of the same age and intelligence – the usual strategy adopted by those examining cognitive deficits in dyslexia? Alternatively, would some other control group be more appropriate? One problem which the age matching procedure encounters is that of 'equating for intelligence'. Dyslexic individuals often obtain a scattered profile of subtest scores on intelligence tests and therefore an aggregate I.Q. score can be an underestimation of ability. Hence, an I.Q. matched control group may not provide a fair comparison, and dyslexic deficits might be underestimated. On the other hand, dyslexic difficulties can be exaggerated if written materials are used in the studies, either as stimuli or as response measures. Vellutino *et al* (1973) found that dyslexics were poorer than aged-matched peers at copying English letter strings but, when both groups were asked to copy an unfamiliar script, namely Hebrew, they were equivalent. Thus, it is always important to ensure that dyslexics and controls are equated in terms of familiarity with the stimuli with which they are asked to deal – otherwise it is tantamount to concluding that dyslexics are poor readers!

Some investigators have avoided the problem discussed above by making use of normal control groups which are matched with the dyslexics in terms of reading experience (or reading age). Unfortunately there are pitfalls in this approach too. The most serious is that, in matching for reading age, dyslexics are immediately allotted a chronological age advantage over their controls. Hence, any processing deficit which caused dyslexia (say at age 6) may no longer be apparent in comparison with a reading age matched control group if dyslexics are tested at age 12. Furthermore, any differences in reading strategy uncovered between the two groups could well be a consequence of the extensive teaching or training which the dyslexics have received. In other words, matching for reading age may reveal the compensatory strategies which the dyslexics have been forced to adopt.

A further problem in this area is concerned with definition of subject groups and indiviudal differences within those groups. Differences between a 'group of dyslexics' and a 'group of normals' could easily be masked if the subjects in each group did not perform in a similar way to each other. This has led some workers to favour an individual case-study approach. Resolution of this issue is beyond the scope of the present chapter. Suffice it to say that the problems of 'group studies' are not so serious in the cases where group differences *are* detected.

There is no one clear-cut solution to these methodological problems and therefore it is vital always to adopt a critical stance when examining the research evidence which exists. In particular, it is important to remember that dyslexia is a developmental disorder; its nature can be expected to change according to the age of the individuals tested and the stage of development they have reached, in whatever domain. Because development is a dynamic process, dyslexics are amenable to training and specific teaching which might 'mask' their underlying pattern of strength and weakness and hide the true reason for their reading failure.

The present chapter will attempt to take account of the above issues when considering an information processing analysis of dyslexia. Discussion will centre upon performance of dyslexic individuals on tasks which are in some cases divorced from reading, with a view to isolating areas in which deficiencies might be apparent as early as the pre-school years and still detectable in adulthood. For discussion of reading and spelling processes in dyslexia, see Snowling, this volume.

The Verbal Deficit Hypothesis

The application of an information processing approach to developmental dyslexia has resulted in a proliferation of theories which aim to account for dyslexia in terms of dysfunction in one, or occasionally more than one, basic process. Vellutino (1979) has undertaken a massive review of the evidence relating to these accounts. Theories which attribute dyslexia to deficiencies in visual perception and memory, deficiencies in intersensory integration or problems with serial order recall have all been considered. Vellutino concluded that there was no clear evidence in favour of any one of these particular accounts. Instead the evidence was interpreted as consistent with a deficit in verbal processing. It was concluded (page 232) that: ' . . . poor readers have deficiencies in both short- and long-term memory characterized by a paucity or inaccessibility of various types of verbal information which would otherwise aid performance on multidimensional tasks by virtue of its coding function.'

There are a number of problems connected with Vellutino's formulation. One of these is that it is too general; it is very difficult to think of a task which has no verbal component to it. Thus, interpretation of a task difference between dyslexics and controls will nearly always be subject to a 'verbal processing' interpretation. A related problem is that the formulation does not specify which verbal processes are impaired in dyslexia and which, if any, are intact. To do so would necessitate specifying what 'verbal processes' are, and investigating them with appropriate experiments. Recent studies have gone some way towards doing this and converging evidence is leading to an understanding of the problems which dyslexics encounter in learning to read. It is to this research evidence which we now turn.

Visual and verbal coding in dyslexia

A popular technique for examining the use of visual and verbal codes is a letter matching task developed by Posner (1969). In this task subjects are shown letter pairs which are either physically identical (AA) or physically distinct (Aa). They are required to respond 'same' to pairs which have the same name and 'different' to pairs which are distinct (AB or Ab). Thus, the task is a 'letter name' matching task. Normal adults can respond 'same' more quickly when letter pairs are physically identical (AA) than when they are physically distinct (Aa). It is assumed that matches can be carried out by reference to a visual code in the case of physically identical pairs but that a verbal code has to be accessed in the latter case.

Using the Posner task, Ellis (1981) found that dyslexic children were slower than age-matched controls when matching physically distinct pairs, but that there was no difference between the groups on the physically identical pairs. The results support the notion that dyslexics have less easy access to a verbal (name) code than normal readers, but are unimpaired in visual matching. Further evidence that dyslexics and controls do not differ in their visual matching abilities comes from two additional studies reported by Ellis (1981). In one study, pairs of shapes were used and 'same' responses were required if the shapes were physically identical. 'Different' responses were required for pairs in which the second member of the pair was a reflected, rotated or mutilated version of the first member of the pair. No differences were found between dyslexics and controls. In a final experiment grids (either 4 by 4 or 5 by 5) were used in which half of the squares of each grid were darkened. Grids were presented in succession with an interval varying from 41-msec to nearly 6 seconds between them. 'Same' responses were required when the two grids were physically identical, 'different' responses were required when the two grids differed by the position of one darkened square. Once again, no differences were found between dyslexics and controls.

In short, dyslexics and controls differed only under conditions which required the use of a verbal, or name, code. There were no differences when the matching could be achieved on a visual basis. Here, then, is one line of evidence which suggests that the nature of the cognitive deficit underlying dyslexia is ease of access to verbal or name codes. In these studies, dyslexics and controls have been matched for age and therefore there is no reason to suspect that either group has been penalized by a developmental disadvantage. The use of letters in the Posner paradigm must be viewed with caution. However, it is important to note that dyslexics were as proficient in dealing with these as controls when the processing which was required was visual in nature.

Access to verbal codes has been assessed more directly in studies which have examined the time taken to name stimuli such as letters, pictures, digits and colours. Spring and Capps (1974) measured the time taken to name 25 line drawings of common objects, the time to name 30 colour patches and the time to name 50 randomly sequenced digits. The results were that dyslexics were slower than controls matched for age and intelligence on all types of materials, the difference between the groups being most pronounced on the digit lists.

Using a similar procedure, Denckla and Rudel (1976a) measured naming times for black and white line drawings of common objects. Dyslexics were found to be slower and also made more naming errors than the control children. In a second study, Denckla and Rudel (1976b) assessed 'Rapid Automatised Naming' of colours, pictures, digits and letters. The stimuli comprised blocks of 50 items made up from a set of five items repeated in random sequences. Error rates were low in this task, however dyslexic children were significantly slower with all four types of stimuli. In addition the dyslexic children were also slower than a second group of non-dyslexic learning disabled children of lower I.Q. It is interesting to note that Denckla and Rudel found naming difficulties with both verbal and visual materials whereas Spring and Capps found that difficulties were more pronounced with verbal materials. A possible age difference between the subjects tested may account for this discrepancy.

Thus the studies which have looked at naming latencies for a variety of materials illustrate that access to a verbal code is slower in dyslexic children than in controls. Interpretation of these studies is not complicated by potential differences in the subjects' experience with text, as would be the case if it were claimed that dyslexics were slower at naming words. However, an alternative interpretation of both the visual matching and the naming studies is that, rather than having poor access to name codes, dyslexics may have difficulty in integrating visual with verbal information. Thus, they may have difficulty in attaching a name code to a visual stimulus, be it pictorial or symbolic. In order to distinguish a deficit in verbal coding from a deficit in visual to verbal recoding, it is important to examine performance in situations where information is presented aurally to dyslexic and normal readers. This is an area which has attracted enormous research attention. We shall consider in detail evidence bearing on the organization and manipulation of auditory information in phoneme segmentation and memory tasks.

Phoneme segmentation

Liberman and Shankweiler have been foremost amongst theorists who have argued that reading ability is closely related to phoneme segmentation skill. The ability to segment the sound stream into phonemic units at an early age is highly predictive of later reading achievement (Liberman and Shankweiler, 1979) and disabled readers are consistently found to be worse than normal readers on tests of phoneme segmentation (Sweeney and Rourke, 1978; Baron *et al*, 1980). The latter finding remains true even if disabled readers are compared with younger normal readers who have reached the same level of reading ability (Bradley and Bryant, 1978). It can be concluded that the dyslexics' segmentation difficulty is not just a consequence of their reading problem but is one of the 'core' characteristics of this group. Furthermore, it is a difficulty which exists independent of visual processing.

The literature on phoneme segmentation in both normally developing and dyslexic readers is extremely varied. The tasks which have been
used to assess segmentation skill include tapping out the individual
sounds in syllables (b + a + t), adding or subtracting phonemes (add s
to lip = slip, take n from bank = back), detecting rhyming relationships
between words (does *hat* rhyme with *cat* or *can*?), finding the odd one
out of four auditorily presented words (sun, sock, *rag*, see), blending
sounds together to give words (c + a + t = cat) and exchanging initial
sounds between two words to make a spoonerism (John Lennon – Lon
Jennon). These tasks vary in terms of how easily they can be
conceptualized, the memory demands which they impose and the types
of response they require as well as in the difficulty of the segmentation
process involved. Thus, it is not easy to pinpoint precisely the reason
for any child's failure. In principle, difficulties with input phonology
(perception), output phonology (production) or phonological memory
could all cause a child to score poorly on segmentation tests.

A number of studies have considered the possibility that dyslexic
children have difficulties at the level of speech perception. Brandt and
Rosen (1980) investigated the discrimination and identification of stop
consonants (e.g. da–ga) by dyslexic and normal readers. The dyslexic
children were not markedly impaired but appeared to be extracting and
encoding phonemic information in a manner characteristic of children
at a younger developmental level. In a more extensive study, Godfrey
et al (1981) found significant differences between dyslexics and controls
(aged 10 years) in both identification and discrimination tasks. Again,
although dyslexics were not grossly abnormal there was inconsistency
in their phonetic classification of auditory cues. In view of this
inconsistency it is worth considering how dyslexics might perform in
situations in which perceptual demands are greater. In classic tests of
speech discrimination, subjects are asked to respond 'same' or
'different' to two auditorily presented items. In tests of phoneme
identification, they are required to decide whether the phoneme they
hear can be categorized as one or other of two prescribed phonemes,
e.g. is it *ba* or *ga*? In both cases, subjects are aware of a finite number of
possible responses and therefore there is considerable redundancy in
the situations. In a more open-ended task dyslexics may be at a greater
disadvantage. For instance, if played a syllable in noise can they
identify it? If told that the letter 'G' says /g/ can they 'hear' it
adequately or will they confuse it with /k/?

A recent study by Brady, Shankweiler and Mann (1983) goes some
way towards answering these questions. They presented good and poor
8-year-old readers with words of high (door, team, road) and low (bale,
din, lobe) frequency for repetition. The words were presented either in
a quiet environment or else with noise masking. The good and poor
readers performed equally well when they were presented with words in
a favourable signal to noise ratio (quiet). Both groups found it easier to
repeat high frequency words, and noise affected performance.
However, of interest was the finding that poor readers made a greater
number of errors than good readers when the words were presented in

noise. Brady *et al* concluded that poor readers require a higher quality signal for error-free performance.

Thus, there are strands of evidence which point to phonemic deficits at the level of speech perception in dyslexic readers. While these difficulties are minor it is worth noting that, at an earlier developmental stage – let's say when the child started school – these difficulties could have been considerably larger in proportion.

An analogous situation obtains when data on speech production deficits in dyslexia are examined. Miles (1973) noted that many dyslexics have difficulty pronouncing polysyllabic words such as 'preliminary' and 'statistical'. However, in his 1983 book, he reminds us that these difficulties must be interpreted in a developmental context. Normal young children cannot be expected to deal with such words, so why should dyslexics? In a similar vein, Snowling (1981) argued that repetition difficulties in dyslexics may be a futher manifestation of their segmentation problem. Dyslexic children were as good as reading age matched readers at repeating real words of two, three and four syllables. However, when asked to repeat nonsense words which were matched with them in terms of phonological complexity (magnificent– bagmivishent), the dyslexic children were worse. Thus, the dyslexics' difficulty cannot be one of articulation *per se* (or else they would have been bad at repeating all of the stimuli). Problems may arise when unfamiliar words have to be processed and segmented in order to set up new articulatory-motor programmes. Of course, at an earlier age, articulation difficulties could have been more noticeable since fewer automatic motor programmes would have been available. Almost by definition, any child who cannot say a word correctly will have difficulty segmenting it at phonemic level.

The present discussion makes clear that it is difficult to separate the skill of phoneme segmentation from other (implicit) phonological processes. Furthermore, explicit segmentation tasks often require that speech stimuli be held in short-term memory and there is ample evidence that dyslexics have verbal memory deficits (see below). There is no doubt that dyslexic children score poorly on segmentation tasks but, as yet, research has not provided a clear picture of why. It is probably the case that different individuals have difficulties for different reasons. What is important for our understanding of dyslexia is that these children have problems with phoneme segmentation at a time when the skill is explicitly required for learning to read, specifically to crack the alphabetic code (Rozin and Gleitman, 1975). Moreover, the problems are specifically *verbal* and quite independent of any visual perceptual process.

Dyslexia and Models of Memory

The two-store model of memory

It is well known that children with specific learning difficulties perform poorly on digit-span tests (Miles, 1983; Rugel, 1974; Thomson, 1982)

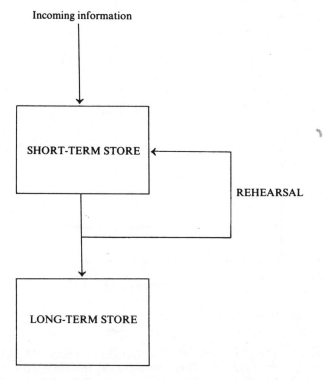

Figure 2.1 Two-store model of memory (after Atkinson and Shiffrin, 1968)

in which sequences of digits have to be repeated, and there is virtual agreement upon deficiencies in other short-term memory tasks. We will consider how these findings can be accommodated by theoretically-based models of memory derived from experimental psychology.

One of the most influential models of memory has been the two-process or two-store model. There are many examples of this class of model, the most typical being that of Atkinson and Shiffrin (1968) (see Figure 2.1). This model regards memory as a two-store system: a short-term store (STS) and a long-term store (LTS), with a rehearsal process which is responsible for maintaining information in the short-term store or transferring it to the long-term store.

Information which is not transferred into long-term store is either displaced by new information or it decays away. One of the strongest pieces of evidence in favour of the two-store model is the 'serial position effect'. If a list of items are presented, the probability of recall for any given item is reliably influenced by the position of that item in the list. A typical serial position curve is shown in Figure 2.2. The superior recall of the first few items (the primacy effect) is thought to reflect retrieval from long-term memory (LTM) – these items have been registered and rehearsed for long-term storage. The superiority of

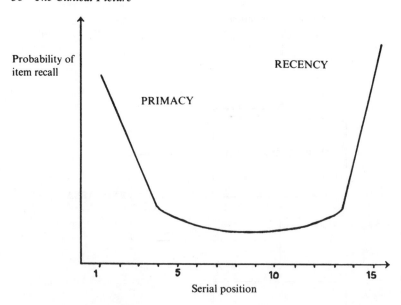

Figure 2.2 Serial position curve

the last few items (the recent effect) is thought to reflect retrieval from short-term memory (STM). These items are still fresh in mind and have not been rehearsed. The middle items are least well remembered. It is assumed that they have not entered long-term memory because rehearsal resources have been used up on the earlier items. Nevertheless they have been displaced from STM because of the arrival of new items.

Spring and Capps (1974) used the Atkinson and Shiffrin model as the basis for an experiment on speech-motor coding and memory. They assumed that rehearsal involves some form of covert speech activity and therefore that the slow speech-motor coding characteristic of dyslexics (and seen in their naming performance) would limit rehearsal in this group. Since rehearsal is the mechanism by which information reaches long-term memory in the two-store model, the primacy effect should be reduced in dyslexic persons. A probed recall technique was used, in which eight cards, each bearing a digit, were shown one by one to the subject and then turned face down in a line. A probe card was then presented and the subjects' task was to point to the card which corresponded to this probe in the line. Each position was probed three times and the number of correct detections at each serial position was recorded. The results showed no group differences with regard to the recency items. The dyslexics remembered the identities of the cards in the final positions as well as controls. However, they recalled fewer of the digits that were presented in the earlier positions and therefore, as predicted, showed a reduced primacy effect.

A more recent study by Bauer and Emhert (1984) examined the effect of rate of presentation on memory in a free recall task. Here, subjects were read a list of words and then asked to write them down in any order. Once again, there was no difference in the recency effect but the dyslexic group showed a reduced primacy effect. Slower presentation increased the primacy effect because it allowed more time for rehearsal, but dyslexics still did not perform as well as controls.

Rehearsal

The process of rehearsal itself has been addressed by a number of studies. In the Spring and Capps (1974) study mentioned above, left to right scanning of the face down memory set was observed upon presentation of the memory probe. This measure of scanning was found to be positively related to memory performance. Bauserman and Obrzut (1981) also attempted to assess the use of rehearsal strategies. In their study, lists of 20 words were presented, each word appearing for one second with a gap of four seconds between words. Subjects were instructed to rehearse the previous items in the gaps following presentation of each word. Two of the measures of rehearsal strategies used were number of different items rehearsed in any one gap, and number of gaps in which a given item was rehearsed. The dyslexic group scored lower on both of these measures and also recalled less items during free recall.

Torgeson and Goldman (1977) investigated the use of rehearsal in an experiment involving memory for order. The subjects were shown pages of a book on which were printed seven pictures of common objects in a different order on each page. The experimenter pointed to a given number of pictures in a predetermined order and the subject then covered his or her eyes for a period of 15 seconds during which period the experimenter noted the number of vocalizations of the object-names and the number of lip-movements or changes of facial expression. (It should be noted that the experimenter was unaware of the reading ability of the children at this stage in the study.) After the 15 second retention interval, the subject was shown the pictures (not in the order seen previously) and required to point to the pictures in the same order as the experimenter had done originally.

It was found that dyslexics verbalized less during the 15 second retention interval and they were also worse at recalling the correct orders. A variation of this experiment was carried out in which the children were required to name the objects during presentation and recall. In this condition there were no differences between the dyslexics and controls in verbalization scores, nor were there differences in order recall.

Torgeson and Goldman interpreted their results as evidence that the dyslexic children fail to use appropriate mnemonic strategies without explicit instruction. They do not speculate as to what might be the basis of this failure. One explanation, consistent with the present discussion, is that the dyslexic children do not have easy access to a name code for the object names. This results in the failure to verbalize and could also account for their poor memory performance. Similarly, it could account for the reduced primacy effect found amongst dyslexics, even when presentation rate is slow. Torgeson and Goldman suggest that the dyslexic children can access a name code when instructed to do so, but that this is not their preferred (or natural) strategy. We will return to the question of the use of alternative codes in a later section. Before then, it is important to consider some studies which have shown that memory differences exist between dyslexic and normal children even in circumstances where rehearsal is not possible.

Cohen and Netley (1981) used a task in which lists of digits were presented auditorily at extremely fast rates of several digits per second. The subject's task was to recall the last three items in each list. However, the lists were of variable length (10 to 26 items) so subjects could not anticipate the to-be-recalled items. Due to the fast rates of presentation and the variable list lengths, Cohen and Netley argued that the use of rehearsal strategies would be unlikely. Dyslexic children were found to recall fewer items than controls and faster rates of presentation decreased performance equally for both groups. The main point to note from the Cohen and Netley study is that memory difficulties were observed in a task demanding rapid auditory processing in circumstances where rehearsal strategies would be unlikely.

Similarly Byrne and Shea (1979) used a monitoring procedure in which subjects listened to a continuous list of words and were required to respond to any word which they had heard earlier in the list. The results showed no overall differences in performance but dyslexic children made more 'false alarm' responses to words which were semantically similar to other words which had been heard earlier (e.g. they responded to TABLE when CHAIR had been heard earlier). In contrast, normal readers made more 'false alarms' to words which sounded similar to words that had been heard previously (e.g. they responded to FAIR when CHAIR had been heard previously). Whilst some rehearsal may have been possible, the nature of the task makes this unlikely. The finding of a larger effect of semantically similar distractors in the dyslexic group is important since it shows that the words were being attended to and processed to a level at which their meanings were available. However, of interest was the finding that the items were being held in a different form to that in which items were stored by the normal readers. It is probable that this difference reflects an encoding difference between the two groups. The dyslexics were utilizing a semantic code for storage while the normal controls were using a phonological (sound based) code.

The findings of this study, together with those of Cohen and Netley (*ibid*) and Bauer and Emert (*ibid*), highlight the inadequacy of theories which attribute the memory deficits in dyslexia to deficiencies in the rehearsal process *per se*. A more parsimonious explanation is that rehearsal is compromised in dyslexics because of inadequate access to verbal, specifically phonological, name codes.

Phonological coding in memory

It is a well established finding that phonological coding is important in short-term memory tasks (Baddeley, 1976). The evidence for its importance originated from studies carried out by Conrad (1964) who presented subjects with sequences of letters which were either phonetically confuseable (BCGTPVD) or were phonetically distinct (HQSLRWK). Subjects were required to repeat the letters which they had heard in the same order as presented by the experimenter. Consistently more errors occurred on the sequences which could be confused phonetically. Later, Baddeley (1966) obtained the same 'phonetic confuseability effect' using sequences of words. These results are usually used as evidence that the type of coding involved in short-term memory is phonological (sound based).

Shankweiler, Liberman, Mark, Fowler and Fischer (1979) have explored the hypothesis that poor readers (dyslexics) fail to use phonetic coding in memory. Following Conrad (1964) they presented groups of normal readers and dyslexics matched for chronological age with sequences of letters for subsequent recall. Normal readers were subject to a 'phonetic confuseability effect.' They made more errors with phonetically confuseable sequences. However, dyslexics showed this effect to a significantly lesser degree, regardless of whether the stimuli were presented auditorily or visually. These findings, in conjunction with those of Byrne and Shea (*ibid*) are consistent with the view that dyslexics are unable to make effective use of a phonological (name) code in memory. In view of the importance of phonetic coding in short-term memory, it would be tempting to suggest that this is the locus of their deficit. Indeed Jorm (1984) has argued for a short-term memory account. However, it will be recalled that the other studies mentioned above have suggested a rehearsal deficit leading to a reduced primacy (LTM) effect. In sum, this would imply that all components of the memory model are impaired. This cannot be the case for, if it were, then dyslexics would experience more widespread (general) learning difficulties.

The levels of processing framework

Craik and Lockhart (1972) proposed an alternative 'model' of memory. They were motivated in part by a dissatisfaction with the notion of rehearsal as the mechanism by which information entered long-term memory. The central feature of their proposal is that memory for an item is largely determined by the type of processing that is applied to that item. Thus, Craik and Tulving (1975) showed that words that had been processed to a semantic level (for example where a category membership judgement had to be made) were recalled better than words that had been processed to a phonological level (where a rhyme judgement was made). These, in turn, were better recalled than words which had been processed to a visual level (for example, where a case judgement was made).

The Craik–Lockhart approach has not been universally accepted (Baddeley, 1978). However, there are a number of useful concepts that have arisen from it, in particular the notion of elaboration. This concept was introduced by Craik and Tulving (1975) who argued that memory for an item would be better the more elaborate the memory trace formed for that item. Nelson and Borden (1977) have argued that this will be so since there are more ways in which recall of the item can be cued. Thus they demonstrated that cues which were both visually and semantically related to target words ('cost' for 'cash') were more effective than cues which were only semantically similar ('price' for 'cash'). To consider an example; suppose you find yourself in a bookshop and you recall that there is a book that you have been meaning to buy. If for some reason you forget the author, you still might locate the book under the title or the publisher. In memory terms, there are a number of ways in which recall of the target might be cued. The more elaborate the memory trace you have, that is the more information which you have stored about the target, the greater the chances of a cue accessing the memory trace and the target being recalled.

In a study by Rack (in press), it was hypothesized that a failure by dyslexics to make use of phonological codes would severely restrict the nature of the memory traces they could form. In particular, dyslexics should not be able to make use of phonetic similarity (rhyme) as a cue for recall. Visual (or orthographic) coding was also investigated since it was considered that dyslexics might utilize an alternative coding system if they were unable to make use of a phonetic code.

In order to investigate these hypotheses, pairs of words were presented to the subjects, who had to decide whether or not the two words rhymed. Four different types of word pair were presented: pairs which rhymed and were orthographically similar (farm–harm), pairs which rhymed but were not similar orthographically (head–said), pairs which were orthographically similar but did not rhyme (low–how) and lastly, control pairs which had neither orthographic nor phonetic similarity (stood–car). Following the rhyme judgement phase of the experiment, subjects were unexpectedly presented with one word from each pair (e.g low) and asked to recall the word which had been presented with it previously (how). The effectiveness of the different types of cue made possible an assessment of the type of coding used by the children.

As expected, normal readers made use of phonetic similarity as a cue for recall; they recalled best words which had been paired with rhyming partners (regardless of orthographic similarity). In contrast, dyslexics (who were equivalent to controls in terms of reading experience) failed to make use of the phonetic similarity between items. Instead they made more use of orthographic similarity as a cue for recall. They remembered best pairs which were orthographically similar, e.g. harm–warm, regardless of phonetic similarity. This finding suggests that the dyslexics were coding words in more of a visually-based form than were controls of the same reading age. With auditory presentation, the dyslexic group was again found to make more use of orthographic similarity as a cue for recall. However, in this case they also made some use of phonetic similarity. It should be noted, with both visual and auditory presentation, that the overall performance of the two groups was similar – they recalled an equivalent number of items. However, the cues which were effective for retrieving these, and by inference the way in whch they were encoded, were different.

The above study is important because it shows that, while dyslexic children do not make as much use of a phonetic code in memory as normal readers, they do have alternative (perhaps compensatory) codes available to them. Thus, their performance in certain memory paradigms may be poor but they do not have a generalized learning difficulty. When processing other than verbal is required, dyslexics do not usually have problems and when memory codes other than phonological can be used, their performance may be unimpaired.

In sum, the evidence for memory deficits in dyslexia is indisputable. However, there is little agreement as to what interpretation to place upon these findings. We have considered evidence in the light of two models of memory. The two-store model is of limited usefulness as deficits have been reported in all three components (STM, rehearsal and LTM). We would be forced to conclude that dyslexics have difficulty with all verbal learning tasks. While plausible, this interpretation leaves us uneasy as it is suggestive of some general slowness or inability to learn. As an alternative, the 'levels of processing' account provides the possibility that dyslexics have difficulty only in specific circumstances, namely whenever a phonological (name) code has to be accessed either to 'elaborate' the memory trace or as a cue to allow successful retrieval of stored information.

Conclusions

We have considered four main areas of research which have investigated cognitive processes in dyslexia. The overwhelming conclusion reached was that dyslexic children experience difficulties in tasks which require verbal, or, more specifically, phonological, processing. It will be recalled that Morrison and Manis (1983) criticize 'deficit' explanations of this kind on three counts. Firstly, they ask why a processing deficit should specifically affect the task of reading. The evidence we have considered comes primarily from tasks divorced from reading; phonological deficits have been found to affect visual matching (in certain circumstances), naming and segmentation processes.

Furthermore, in memory tasks which require the use of a phonological code, dyslexics have been shown to be impaired.

Secondly, Morrison and Manis (1983) consider it important to specify the mechanism by which reading acquisition is affected. It goes without saying that reading involves the association of visual and verbal symbols. We have seen from the work on visual matching that dyslexics do not have a specific difficulty in visual processing. Therefore it is unlikely to be the visual demands of reading which cause failure. One possible explanation is that dyslexics are impaired in their ability to access name codes; we have seen that they are slower in naming tasks than normal readers. Since reading involves accessing verbal labels from long-term memory, it could be this process which is at fault. In addition, and perhaps of more serious consequences for those learning to read, dyslexics have difficulties with phoneme segmentation. These difficulties hinder the understanding of letter–sound relationships and the alphabetic principle.

Finally, with regard to the causality issue, it would be difficult to argue that the phonological deficits we have seen are simply a consequence of reading failure in dyslexia. The deficits can be seen in auditory processing tasks even when dyslexics are compared with younger controls who are reading at the same level as they are. Furthermore, the deficits are potentially identifiable in the pre-reader and persist into adulthood. Indeed, the specific nature of the deficit is such that associated problems will differ according to the age and experience of the child. In particular, the demands of learning to read change over time. In the early stages, reading is visually based and the dyslexics' difficulties may be relatively small. Later, when phonological skill is required for reading (and spelling) the dyslexics' difficulty will be pronounced. However, this does not mean that development will be completely arrested. Alternative compensatory strategies may be available – research shows that dyslexics can learn to read by relying heavily upon visual strategies (Snowling, 1980). In memory too, there is evidence that dyslexics may use alternative codes (visual, semantic or kinaesthetic) where phonetic coding fails (Rack, in press).

In sum, we have seen that dyslexia is a specific developmental disorder. By considering it in processing terms, it has been possible to identify efficient as well as deficient skills. Information processing models which elucidate those components common to memory and reading are needed. The evidence we have discussed goes some way towards developing such a model and future research might usefully be guided by these considerations.

Peter Bryant

3 The Question of Prevention

No one could complain that dyslexic children have not received their fair share of attention, at any rate from psychologists, paediatricians, teachers and child psychiatrists. How many dyslexics are there? What is their background? What's wrong with them? How do we teach them? These are questions which, if not actually on everyone's lips, are on enough lips to give the condition a noticeable presence in journals and books on child development and on education. And it has not been in vain. There is no doubt that the last ten years have seen great strides made towards knowing what ought to be known about these unfortunate children.

However, in all the experimental studies, case histories and epidemiological surveys which make up this lively endeavour, one topic has been sadly neglected. It is the simple and startlingly obvious question of prevention. How can we stop the problem in the first place? What steps should we take, long before children go to school, in order to make sure that those who run the risk of becoming dyslexic never succumb to this unworthy fate? There are endless studies whose aim it is to discover the 'deficit' responsible for the problem. We know now how well many remedial teaching programmes work with these children, but there is nothing to tell us how to make sure that a child – any child – will have picked up all the necessary skills by the time he goes to school to avoid becoming a dyslexic.

Yet the question itself cannot be faulted. It would surely be a much better thing to prevent the problem than to wait until it happens and only then, after a history of frustration and feelings of failure on the part of the child, to step in and try and do something about it. Moreover in principle it seems to me to be quite probable that there *are* some specific steps which one could take when children are three or four years old and which would make sure that they do not follow a course of development that would end in dyslexia. After all, most of the theories about the problem are based on the assumption that there is some highly specific cause and if that is so, it ought to be possible to do something about it early on in the child's life.

If the central question about prevention is such a good one (and a practicable one at that), why then have so few people tried to answer it? I think that one apparent stumbling block has been responsible for this worrying gap. The argument that I shall develop in this chapter is that 'apparent' is exactly the right word. It is not a *real* block. There never has been any need to stumble nor any good reason for people to keep so well away from the question of prevention.

Who are Dyslexic Children?

Before I describe the block, I must make it clear what I mean by another term – the term 'dyslexia'(By this I mean exactly the same as Rutter and Yule (1975) meant when they wrote about 'specific reading retardation'. They pointed out that many children fall well behind their peers when learning to read, but that this is only surprising in some cases. Many of these children are generally behind in everything and characteristically have a low I.Q. Their relative failure in learning to read is certainly distressing and steps should be taken to help them, but it is just one failure among many and, in this way, not at all surprising. There is a strong relationship between I.Q. and reading – so strong in fact that it is possible to make a pretty accurate estimate of how well most children can read from their intelligence test scores. These generally backward children are not on the whole exceptions. Their poor reading is only to be expected from their low I.Q.

On the other hand there are children – 'specific reading retardates' to use Rutter and Yule's words or 'dyslexics' if you prefer the shorter term – whose difficulties in reading are a real surprise. These children are blatant exceptions to the strong relationship between intelligence and success in reading. Their I.Q. scores lead you to expect them to reach one level in reading: reading tests show them to be at quite another, and much lower, level. Notice that these children do not have to be particularly bright or even of average intelligence to qualify as dyslexics. They simply have to be exceptional in the sense that their reading scores fall well below what one would expect from their general intelligence.

There is of course no dispute that such children do exist and epidemiological studies agree that their numbers are high (Rutter and Yule, 1975; Yule *et al*, 1974; Rodgers, 1983). Whether they constitute a homogeneous group is another, more controversial, matter. So is the question of what precisely leads to their surprising problems, and so too is the subject of the right teaching method. But these at least are questions on which people do research. What about the neglected question – prevention?

Prediction – the stumbling block

We can at least rephrase the question, now that we know whom we are discussing. Among our pre-school children there are some who will eventually flout everyone's expectations and do very much worse at learning to read than one would predict, given their general abilities.

This is unless something is done about it before they begin to be taught to read. But here we come to the difficulty which I suspect has put most people off 'doing something about it'.

The problem is this. If everyone expects these children to read reasonably well, no one is going to know about their problem before they begin to be taught to read. So, 'doing something about it' means helping these children *before* they are known to have a problem. But that at first seems to be impossible. How can we go out and help these children before they begin to learn to read, when we have no way of knowing who they are? This then is the apparent stumbling block.

There is a more technical way of putting this. The question of prevention seems, at first sight, to be inextricably linked with the question of prediction. It looks as though there is no point in anyone trying to prevent children ever becoming dyslexic without having a precise way of detecting exactly which child among a group of three or four year olds is likely to do much worse at learning to read than would be expected from his or her general intelligence. Otherwise, we would end up taking preventative steps with children who don't – and ignoring others who desperately do – need this sort of help.

The trouble is, however, that no such measure exists. There is no precise way of establishing, years before children go to school, who among them will fall below the expected level of reading. We can always have quite a confident stab at spotting the ones who will fall behind in reading and in everything else by picking out those with low I.Q. and verbal skills. But generally backward children are not what we are talking about at the moment. We are looking for a test which will say who will do *worse* at reading than his I.Q. or verbal skills would lead us to expect, and as far as I know no such test exists. There have been several attempts to find one, but no one has produced one which makes certain, or even reasonably certain, predictions about which particular pre-school child will fall behind the reading level which normally goes with their I.Q.

Predictive studies

This might at first seem surprising to anyone who has a passing acquaintance with work on this topic. Surely there have been quite a few predictive studies, and surely, too, some of these have had positive results? This is certainly true. There have been some decent longitudinal studies – not enough, but some at any rate – which have involved large groups of children and have shown that measures taken some time before these children go to school are related to how well they read, *independently* of how intelligent they are (see, for example, the Swedish study by Lundberg, Olofsson and Wall, 1981). There is a definite relationship between these pre-school measures and the extent to which children involved do better or worse than would be expected given their overall level of intelligence. The lower they come on the screening measure in question, the more likely it is that their reading will fall below expectation. So why shouldn't these measures be used universally to pick out the three and four year olds who run a definite risk of becoming dyslexic in a few years' time?

The answer unfortunately is that there is a very great difference between an overall relationship, a correlation, of the sort found in these studies and a test which makes really accurate predictions about individual people. You can get a picture of the overall relationship and still not have anything like an accurate enough tool, precise enough to dig out the right individuals.

As an example let me use a longitudinal study carried out recently by Lynette Bradley and myself (Bradley and Bryant, 1983; 1985). This was successful by its own lights but never came near to producing a measure which made really accurate and confident predictions about individual children. The study was about the importance of children's awareness of sounds in words. In order to be able to understand the way the alphabet works the child must realize that words and syllables can be broken up into smaller units of sound and it is a fair bet that the basis for that understanding is laid down sometime before children go to school. For example, when a child listens to rhymes and produces them himself – a commonplace in many pre-school children's lives – he is breaking up words in just this way. To know that 'cat' and 'hat' rhyme is to realize that they have a sound in common, and that recognition must indicate some inkling in the child that these words consist of a number of different sounds that are able to be separated.

In order to see whether this was so, in the study we gave a large group (just over 400 of them) of four- and five-year-old children, none of whom could yet read, tests of their ability to detect rhyme and alliteration. They had to work out which of the three or four words that we read out to them did not rhyme with the rest or did not start with the same sound. We also gave them a number of other tests at this time including tests of memory and of vocabulary. Then we followed the same children's progress over the next three to four years. We looked at their progress in learning to read and to spell and in mathematics, and we also measured their intelligence. (In addition to this we included an element of training: we taught some children to categorize words by their sounds and other children to categorize them in other different ways.)

Our results were very positive. There was a strong and highly significant relationship between the children's scores on our original measures of awareness of rhyme and alliteration and their progress in reading and spelling (but not in mathematics) even when the effects of the children's intelligence had been controlled. This meant that our measures were related to the degree to which children departed from expectation. On the whole children who did poorly on our original tests of rhyme and alliteration also fell below expectation in reading. Our belief that this showed that awareness of the sounds in words is one of the causes of progress in reading was bolstered because we also found that teaching these children how to categorize words by sounds did definitely improve their reading.

So far, so good. An overall relationship – independent of intelligence – between our pre-school measures and reading does exist and is important. But what about accurate predictions about individual children? Here we have quite a different tale to tell.

Individual predictions – the stumbling block

We wanted to know whether unusual scores in our original tests would predict success or failure in learning to read. However, put as directly as this, the question is altogether too simple. Obviously there are children who will do remarkably badly or well on any test (sound categorization included) and will do particularly badly or well when it is time for them to learn to read. These children's success or failure would be predicted at least as well by other measures, such as tests of I.Q. or of verbal skills. If this were all, measures of sound categorization would not add anything to our ability to predict success or failure.

Instead our question was would any child whose sound categorization scores are unusually poor (or unusually good), *after both his vocabulary and his age at the time of the initial tests are taken into account,* learn to read and to spell unusually unsuccessfully (or unusually well) *after his I.Q. has been taken into account.* We used the relation (the regression) between children's vocabulary and their scores on our sound categorization tests to decide which children among the group were particularly weak (or good) in our initial tests of sound categorization. They were classified as weak if their scores on these tests fell well below the level that would be expected from their vocabulary. In just the same way, we used the relation (the regression) between reading or spelling and I.Q. to decide who were the children who had turned out in the end to be considerably worse (or better) at reading than expected. In our view, these children were unusual if their reading or spelling scores diverged quite a bit from the level to be expected from their age and I.Q. (If the child was one standard deviation or more above or below his expected sound categorization or his reading and spelling score, we treated him as exceptionally good or bad at this particular skill. Similarly if his reading or spelling scores were one standard deviation away from the level that would have been expected from his age and from his I.Q., we treated him as a good or a poor reader/speller.)

Then we looked to see whether exceptionally good sound categorizers would end up as exceptionally skilled readers/spellers, and exceptionally poor sound categorizers vice versa. Table 3.1 shows how many of the children who had proved to be exceptionally weak or exceptionally good in the initial sound categorization tests went on to become unexpectedly poor or good readers.

The table shows that less than a third of our unusually good sound categorizers went on to become unusually good readers and less than a third of our poor sound categorizers ended up as unusually weak readers, at any rate as far as reading measured by the Neale reading test

	Percentage of children one S.D. above expected sound categorization scores	Percentage of children one S.D. below expected sound categorization scores
Unexpectedly high readers	30.18	5.66
Unexpectedly low readers	4.00	28.00

Table 3.1 Percentage of unexpectedly high and low scorers on initial sound categorization tests who became unexpectedly good and poor readers (Neale)

is concerned. So, with this measure at least, we now know that our sound categorization tests on their own will not be a very precise predictor of success or failure in reading. We certainly cannot be certain than an individual child who does very well on our sound categorization tests, or likewise very poorly, will turn out to be an exceptional reader. Less than a third of them do.

This is only one test. However our other reading test goes much the same way. Tables 3.2 and 3.3 show much the same pattern with the Schonell reading and spelling test scores.

	Percentage of children one S.D. above expected sound categorization scores	Percentage of children one S.D. below expected sound categorization scores
Unexpectedly high readers	32.08	5.66
Unexpectedly low readers	4.00	24.00

Table 3.2 Percentage of unexpectedly high and low scorers on initial sound categorization tests who became unexpectedly good and poor readers (Schonell)

Our three tests of reading/spelling tell a consistent story. Roughly a quarter to a third of those who produced unusual scores in the sound categorization test became exceptional readers or spellers. So, on its own, our test will not be much use at predicting success or failure in reading and spelling. Its scores will not show with any degree of certainty whether individual children will eventually experience learning difficulties.

	Percentage of children one S.D. above expected sound categorization scores	Percentage of children one S.D. below expected sound categorization scores
Unexpectedly high spellers	28.30	3.77
Unexpectedly low spellers	0.00	28.00

Table 3.3 Percentage of unexpectedly high and low scorers on initial sound categorization tests who became unexpectedly good and poor spellers (Schonell)

Perhaps we should not be surprised. We had after all set ourselves a very difficult task, since we were trying to make not the crude prediction of who would become poor readers, but the much more sophisticated prediction of who would read below the level predicted by their I.Q. We set ourselves against I.Q. and tried to predict reading skills despite it. Nobody as far as we know has managed to do that at all successfully, and we, it must be said, have had a modicum of success.

The proportion of children who (on our measures) were weak sound categorizers and went on to become poor readers/spellers was far higher than the proportion of children whose sound categorization scores were within one standard deviation of their expected score. For example, 28.57 per cent of our weak sound categorizers went on to become weak readers too by our 'Neale' measure (i.e. one standard deviation or more below what would have been expected from their I.Q. score), whereas only 15.54 per cent of those whose sound categorization scores were within one standard deviation of their expected level became backward readers. The equivalent figures for the Schonell reading test were respectively 24.00 per cent versus 16.80 per cent and for the Schonell spelling test 28.00 per cent versus 17.64 per cent. So even at their weakest point as predictors our sound categorization measures do better than no measures at all.

Nevertheless, these measures are plainly not good enough for anyone interested in prevention who insists on an accurate measure for predicting which child definitely risks becoming dyslexic, and since there do not seem to be any better predictors than these in the market, we can understand why people have been so deterred from trying to take the path of 'prevention'.

Does this indicate that we have to abandon the attempt? Only, I think, if one accepts the demand for an accurate predictor. Is it really so important that we should know who is likely to turn into a dyslexic? The answer is that it is important only if one makes the assumption that there are qualitative differences between dyslexic children and others. If that assumption, which many people do make, is correct, then dyslexic children will need special forms of teaching: these should help them but will probably not be much benefit to anyone else. In that case we really do need to know who these children are, because otherwise we will waste our time teaching the wrong children. What helps a dyslexic child would be of no use to another.

But suppose that this assumption were not true. Suppose instead that there were no qualitative differences between dyslexic children and others, and that the only differences were quantitative ones. Suppose that dyslexic children are affected by the same forces as other children when they learn to read, that they learn in exactly the same way – only slower, and call on exactly the same skills – but have less of them. In that case, what would help the dyslexic child would also help every other child. If we think again about prevention and the question of what one does to prepare pre-school children for reading, any method that would prepare a child who risks becoming dyslexic would also prepare other children as well.

In other words, there would be no necessity for an accurate predictor. On the contrary, one could with relief abandon any idea of selection at all, because the same experiences would help all children – potentially dyslexic and normal children alike – which is an obviously worthwhile aim.

The Question of the Continuum

Everything thus seems to turn on the question of qualitative versus quantitative differences between dyslexic children and the rest, and here we find ourselves on a decidedly well trodden path. The topic, when it comes up, is usually known as the question of the continuum. Many people have raised it. Are dyslexic children simply at the wrong end of a continuum of ability which determines how well their progress in reading accords with expectation? Or is there some radical difference between these children and the rest which would mean that they set about reading in an entirely different way and therefore need, as we have seen, entirely different kinds of teaching?

I should like to declare my hand at this stage. I believe in the continuum. It seems to me that all the signs point to their being a quantitative but no qualitative difference between dyslexic and other children; that dyslexic children learn to read in the same way, only slower; that they make the same kind of mistakes, only more of them. All of this is because they call on the same skills to learn to read but happen to possess them to a much smaller degree than other children. But having stated this view, I must immediately own that it is an unpopular one. Most of the people directly concerned with the question of dyslexia insist on qualitative differences and reject the idea of a continuum.

Let us turn to their reasons for doing this. Broadly speaking, there are three types of evidence that have been used to support the idea of there being qualitative differences between dyslexic children and the rest. One is epidemiological and consists of studies of thousands of children. The second type comes from direct comparisons between groups of dyslexic and of normal children and the third involves intensive studies of individual dyslexic children.

Epidemiological studies and the continuum

The most famous epidemiological study of children's reading dif-ficulties – and the one most often used to support the idea of a discontinuity between poor readers and the others – is the Isle of Wight study (Yule *et al*, 1974). This involved all the nine- and ten-year-old children on the Isle. Among other things, measures were taken of their intelligence and their reading ability. As usual, there was a strong correlation between these two measures: the more intelligent the children, the better on the whole their progress in reading. The research team then used this relationship to work out how well individual children were reading *vis à vis* what would be expected from their I.Q. It was no surprise that though most children read nearly as well as would be expected from their I.Q., there were several who diverged quite markedly from expectation, some doing better and others worse.

However, these divergences took a somewhat singular form. When the research team looked at the extreme divergences (those who had done very much better and those who had done very much worse at reading than expected) they found that there were more of the latter kind – extreme failures in reading – and many more than would be expected if these divergences had been normally distributed. So the research team argued for the existence of a special group or groups (they did not claim to have found a homogeneous group) of 'specific reading retardates'. This claim has often been used to support the notion that dyslexic children do not just fall at the lower end of the continuum of reading skill but that they have problems of their own idiosyncratic kind.

There are problems, however. One is that there is now some conflicting evidence. A recent paper by Rodgers (1983) on a study of a very large number of ten year olds reports no such pattern. He found exactly the same number of children diverging sharply from expectation in both directions – an entirely normal distribution of divergences. In fact there were slight differences in his method (the Isle of Wight team had tested non-verbal I.Q. whereas Rodgers tested total I.Q.), but in my opinion the contradiction is almost certainly due to the fact that Rodgers used a different and more satisfactory reading test. The Isle of Wight reading test suffered from the fact that it was too easy: many children got 100 per cent correct scores and still did not count as particularly good readers for their I.Q.: they would have had to have a score over 100 per cent for that (an impossibility). It is quite likely that the peculiar Isle of Wight pattern can be traced back to that unfortunate fact. So we must conclude that if anything the epidemiological evidence that we have supports the notion of the continuum.

Group comparisons, the mental age match, and the continuum

Group studies also have their problems. There must be thousands of these and the vast majority take the same form; a form which I shall refer to as the 'mental age match'. The researcher has a theory about some oddity in the psychological make up of dyslexic children – let's say that they cannot think of the right word when they see something and therefore have difficulty in thinking of the right spoken word when they see its written version. So a group of ten-year-old dyslexic children is gathered together, children who read at the level of a typical seven year old, and likewise a group of normal ten-year-old children who read at the ten-year-old level. Both groups are normal in intelligence and thus have the same mental age. The researcher then tests the speed with which the children come up with the names of familiar objects, colours and numbers. If the dyslexic group is slower, it is argued that you have found a genuine difference between them and the rest. (In fact an experiment rather like this, but involving several age groups, was done by Denckla and Rudel (1976).)

Experiments which take exactly this form have been used at different times to establish claims of a verbal deficit in dyslexic children (Vellutino, 1979), a memory deficit (Jorm, 1983), a 'decoding deficit' (Perfetti and Hogaboam, 1975) and a deficit in linking vision with hearing (Birch and Belmont, 1964). In fact, they form the basis for most claims for qualitative differences between dyslexic children and the rest. And yet such claims are worthless.

The trouble lies in a confusion between cause and effect. Without any doubt the experience of reading will have its effect on children. Reading introduces children to new kinds of information presented in a new kind of way. Normal readers will have had much more of this experience than dyslexic children of the same age. It follows that any differences that emerge in the 'mental age match' kind of study may be the result rather than the cause of the reading difficulty. But we are looking for causes and not results. We want to know what determines a dyslexic child's difficulties. So, for this reason, all the results from this kind of comparison must remain completely ambiguous.

Group comparisons, the reading age match, and the continuum

Is there a solution? Recently another kind of comparison between groups of dyslexic and normal children has been tried; this is the 'reading age match'. In this case a group of, say, ten-year-old dyslexic children who have a reading age of 7 are compared with a seven-year-old group of normal children with the same reading age. Both groups have reached the same level of reading and so any difference that is found between them cannot be due to a difference in reading levels.

It is still early days yet, but the signs are that studies of this kind have produced one consistent and strong difference between dyslexic children and others. This is in the awareness of sounds in words, i.e. in 'phonological awareness'. One way of measuring this awareness is to give children nonsense words to read, words like 'slosbon'. It is a fair assumption that in order to read words as completely unfamiliar as these are, children will have to call on their knowledge of letter–sound correspondences. It is now clear from studies by Frith and Snowling (1983) and by Baddeley et al (1982) (see also a paper by Snowling, 1980) that this is something which dyslexic children find very difficult to do. The above were all 'reading age match' studies and they showed that although the dyslexic and normal children read real words as well as each other (no surprise this, since they were at the same level of reading), the dyslexic children were much worse when it came to the nonsense words.

Another reason for thinking that dyslexic children might be insensitive to sounds in words is a reading age match study done some time ago (1978) by Lynette Bradley and myself which compared ten-year-old dyslexic children with a reading age of 7 to normal children with the same reading age. We looked at their ability to detect rhyme and alliteration, using exactly the same kind of task which I described earlier and we found that the dyslexic children made many more mistakes. They are much worse at categorizing words by sounds. Here then is a genuine difference.

However, does this sort of result mean that there is no continuum? Does it mean that dyslexic children suffer from some idiosyncratic difficulty which adds up to a qualitative difference between themselves and others? In my view, it does not. In fact, I think that it means the exact opposite.

Let us put the last result (dyslexic children worse at detecting rhyme) together with the result which I mentioned earlier on, which was that in general children's skills at detecting rhyme are related to how well they learn to read, independent of intelligence. This means that the connection between detecting rhyme and reading is not something confined to the dyslexic child's difficulties. The connection holds right through the continuum. Not only are children who are poor at detecting rhyme also worse on the whole at reading than would be expected from their I.Q. It is also the case that children who are good at detecting rhyme will on the whole do better in reading than expected. In other words, dyslexic children are simply at one end – the wrong end – of a continuum which stretches from where they stand right through to spectacularly good readers at the other end.

As far as I know, the difference in phonological awareness is the only consistent result to emerge from reading age match studies. I conclude therefore that group comparisons end up supporting the notion of a continuum.

Individual cases and the continuum

We come now to the third major type of evidence about differences between dyslexic children and others – the detailed study of individual cases of dyslexia. Those who are most insistent that backward readers are a separate and distinctive group of children are often the parents, remedial teachers or psychologists who have had a great deal of contact with individual backward readers. People who get to know dyslexic children are so struck by their peculiarities that they conclude that there must be something distinctive about them.

This kind of conviction that dyslexic children are distinctively different has been most clearly embodied in research by recent studies which make a connection between 'developmental' and 'acquired' dyslexia. 'Acquired dyslexia' refers to adults who originally had no problem about learning to read, but who later, because of some kind of damage to their brain, either lost their ability to read or at least found it a great deal more difficult than before. Acquired dyslexics do form a distinct group. They have something in common (damage to their brain) which other people do not have, or at any rate do not have so severely. They are not a homogeneous group: there are different forms of acquired dyslexia. One is 'phonological dyslexia'. It involves difficulties with the analysis of sounds. 'Phonological dyslexics' have difficulty reading nonsense words and they make mistakes which suggest that they are leaning heavily on the visual appearance of the word. These mistakes are called derivational errors ('weigh' read as 'weight') and visual errors ('camp' read as 'cape'). Phonological dyslexics seem to use the visual appearance of words and perhaps their orthographic sequences as well, rather than analysing them into phonological segments.

There is yet another form of acquired dyslexia called 'surface dyslexia'. 'Surface dyslexics' seem to be alright as far as their phonological skills are concerned. They read and write nonsense words reasonably well. Their difficulty is with words which one cannot read simply with the help of letter–sound correspondences. These people find it very difficult to remember and to read irregular words. Another of their difficulties is that they muddle the meaning of homophones – words like 'bear' and 'beer', or 'soar' and 'saw', which sound much the same but mean quite different things. So the surface dyslexic finds it difficult to remember what words look like and depends too heavily on working out the words' meanings through rules about letter–sound relationships.

These two forms of acquired dyslexia have been the inspiration for a number of recent detailed descriptions of individual dyslexic children. The idea behind these studies has been that developmental dyslexics may be like acquired dyslexics (Ellis, 1984). If it is true that there are some children with reading difficulties who read in the same way as phonological dyslexics and others who are exactly like surface dyslexics, then here surely would be evidence that 'dyslexia' in children is a distinctive condition.

One example of this kind of study is by Temple and Marshall (1983). In this work, an intelligent seventeen-year-old girl was studied. Her reading and spelling skills at the time were around the nine-and ten-year-level and she had always had difficulties with written language. This girl looked like an adult phonological dyslexic. She was bad at reading nonsense words, made 'derivational' and 'visual' errors ('height' for 'high' and 'achieve' for 'attractive') and stumbled over long but regular words, like 'herpetology', which can in principle be read by using letter–sound rules.

At first the case looks convincing. But the trouble is that there is no guarantee that the mistakes that this girl made were odd, *given her reading level of 10 years*. Ten-year-old children too make mistakes with nonsense words and long regular words. The girl's difficulties could only be called idiosyncratic if they are not to be found in normal ten-year-old children and there is nothing here to tell us whether or not this is so.

The same problem bedevils an attempt by Coltheart, together with several other colleagues (1983), to link developmental with acquired dyslexia. Their analogy is with surface dyslexia and concerns a girl of sixteen and a half, of average intelligence but seriously behind in reading and spelling: she read at the level of a typical nine to ten year old. She found regular words easier to read than irregular words such as 'gauge' and 'debt'. She was not at all happy with the words which transgressed normal spelling rules. Another similarity between her and the typical surface dyslexic was that she often read words in slightly the wrong way ('beer' for 'bear').

Is this a developmental surface dyslexic? We must hesitate because again we have no guarantee that the girl's mistakes were idiosyncratic. The most striking thing about this girl's reading – her difficulty with irregular words – is something which can be found in the vast majority of children, with and without reading problems (Robertson, 1984).

Recently Lawrence Impey and I gathered together a group of ten-year-old children, none of them backward readers. We gave them the bulk of the tests which both sets of experimenters referred to above had given to each of their children. We found that neither of the two dyslexic children in the studies which I have just described was particularly untypical. We found that the average child in our group made the same sort of mistakes, and just as many of them, as did the 'surface dyslexic' studied by Coltheart and his colleagues. She had no more difficulty than they, on average, did with irregular words and made no more 'regularization' errors than they did on average.

When we compared the same children to Temple and Marshall's 'phonological dyslexic' we found that they made the same kind of mistakes – visual paralexias, derivational errors, nonsense words more difficult to read than real ones – as she. But she made more such mistakes than our children did on average. However, a few of our children were exactly like her: they had the same amount of difficulty with nonsense words, and made the same number of derivational errors and produced the same number of visual paralexias. Thus our study shows that normal children as well as dyslexic children do vary: some read in different ways than others. It looks as though there may be the same sorts of differences among children at every level of reading. That is interesting, but it is a long way from establishing the existence of a group of children at the bottom of the reading ladder whose mistakes are bizarre and unique. On the contrary, our evidence suggests once again the existence of a continuum.

Prevention and the continuum

With this conclusion we can come back to the question of prevention. In the course of this chapter I have reached two conclusions.

One is that there is no evidence at all that dyslexic children constitute a distinct, qualitatively different group (or groups) with their own idiosyncratic problems and their own odd ways of setting about reading and writing. On the contrary all the evidence, once it has been looked at critically, leads to the opposite conclusion. It seems very much as though there is a continuum, and that the children whom we call dyslexic are at the bottom of it.

This, from the point of view of the original question of prevention, is an important *and encouraging* conclusion. It means that we no longer have to worry about selection or accurate prediction before thinking seriously about prevention. It does not matter that we do not and probably never will have accurate enough tools to tell us long before children go to school who precisely will turn out to be a dyslexic. If there is no qualitative difference between these and other children, then what will help them will help everyone. So we just help them all.

But how do we do that? There are probably many ways, but at the moment the best single answer can be found in my second main conclusion, which is that one of the main causes of how well a child reads is his skill with sounds in words. On the whole (though there will be exceptions), if he is good with sounds his reading will surpass expectations and if he is not his reading will fall below those expectations.

But this is a skill which can be fostered and improved in young children. A wealth of evidence shows this (Bradley and Bryant, 1983; Branwhite, 1983; Fox and Routh, 1976; Gittelman and Feingold, 1983; Goldstein, 1976; Olofsson and Lundberg, 1983; Williams, 1980). It is also something that pre-school children enjoy. They revel in nursery rhymes, and they take up their own poems (Chukovsky, 1963). Here then is an activity which happens naturally and informally but which might well have enormous repercussions years later on when the child begins to read. Surely we should concentrate on encouraging it? There is every reason for thinking that by doing so we should be taking a definite step towards the eradication of dyslexia before it ever develops.

Part 2

Procedures for the Assessment and Management of Children with Reading and Spelling Difficulties

Hanna Klein

4 The Assessment and Management of Some Persisting Language Difficulties in the Learning Disabled

The literature relating to children and adolescents with specific learning disability has for many years urged us to take account of the language disorders which *underlie* reading and writing disorders (Johnson and Myklebust, 1967; Wiig and Semel, 1976; Luria, 1966; Wren, 1983; The Bullock Report, 1975). Indeed, Vellutino (Myklebust, 1983, p.135) has stated that impairment in one or more aspects of linguistic development is the probable cause of dyslexia or specific reading disability. (See also Vellutino, 1979.)

Undoubtedly, many complex factors underlie language skills, and the normal acquisition of the mother tongue by the pre-school child may be delayed by a multiplicity of these. However, the concern of this chapter is that the verbal skills needed by the pre-school and the school-going child are very different. The child at school should have integrated all the rules of oral language by the time he enters the classroom. Thereafter, he should be able to attend to, assimilate and create complex abstract language forms which enable him to manipulate his environment in a satisfactory manner (Luria, 1966; Wallach and Butler, 1984.)

If the sophisticated skills of reading, writing and mathematics are superimposed on a faulty base of *oral* language, then pupils may fail to respond appropriately to formal instruction at school. It is always important for a language therapist to screen a child with specific learning disabilities *before* he commences remedial intervention to ensure that his formal language functions are within normal limits. If he fails to perform appropriately on the tasks of linguistic competence, integration or performance, a course of language therapy should at least parallel, if not precede, reading therapy (Alley and Deshler, 1979; Butler, 1984).

The comprehension, integration and expression of language are inextricably linked and an attempt to compartmentalize them may lead to myopic assessments and limited treatment programmes. However, division of test material into categories is essential for a time saving assessment of the child in the first instance when parents are anxious to have some idea of the extent of their child's difficulties. So it is with reluctance that this chapter is divided into sections relating to the 'understanding' and 'production' of language.

Note

('He' is used throughout the chapter for the sake of economy and also because more boys are referred for language therapy than girls. 'Mother' is used where 'father' is as important. 'Child' is used where 'adolescent' may equally apply. Sadly, we see too many adolescents who ought to have received language therapy as primary school children but who were not tested for the more complex, yet subtle, language deficits which we suspect underlie specific learning difficulties.)

The Assessment and Treatment Procedure

Every learning disabled child presents with a different cluster of symptoms, and, although we begin our assessment with a formal test battery, we should then modify our examination to determine individual variation in detail. Since many of the tests which successfully alert us to the presence of linguistic deficit in the learning disabled are designed and standardized in America, the vocabulary and norms of these items may not be valid for use outside the United States. For this reason the procedures described here have been taken from a variety of tests, and results are qualified rather than quantified. Every child's strength and weakness in each sphere of linguistic functioning should be discussed with parents and teachers and realistic recommendations given to help the child reach his maximum potential.

The items presented here are only *some* of the ways in which we may investigate and treat language disorders in children with specific learning disability who, in the first instance, are referred for poor school skills. Treatment is individually designed and frequently altered, depending on the needs of the child in relation to his schoolroom, the playground and his family.

To illustrate this, Alex was referred by his teacher at the age of seven for reading and spelling therapy. He had no history of eye or ear disorders. He spoke late, but no help was sought. His mother complained that he did not listen to her, but she felt there was nothing wrong with his language since he spoke a great deal. She was very surprised to discover that his receptive vocabulary, his short-term auditory memory, and his comprehension of verbal material were below age level. He had a severe expressive word-finding difficulty. Before we could begin to teach him how to read and spell to age level, we tried to upgrade his overall oral language function. An interesting example of his comprehension difficulties arose during one session when we were using the Galt 'How To Measure' game. Alex was asked to read the card which said: 'How wide is the gate?'. He read this phrase correctly, but placed the blocks from one end of the gate to the other end of the card. After two verbal 'translations' of the instruction, Alex completed the task correctly. He then had to read and complete the next card: 'How long is the train?'. He did this correctly, but placed the blocks in a line on the train, rather than between the two black lines designed to hold the blocks, He could not however answer the question: 'How much longer is the train than the gate?' It was of interest that he could complete the sum: $10 - 3 = 7$, which was the numerical representation of the verbal problem he was unable to solve. As his mother looked on, it seemed that she had begun to understand the extent of Alex's problems for the first time.

In clinical practice it has been very useful to encourage parents to sit in the room to observe testing and treatment. In this way the child's family can be alerted to his pattern of functioning, where no amount of 'telling them' could have the same effect. Progress appears much more rapid in those children whose parents and teachers actively participate in the treatment programme. It is interesting how dedicated they are to the practice of new skills at home and in the classroom. Since diagnosis ends only when therapy ends, we should pay close attention to the child during each session and should dovetail the lesson to each emerging strength and weakness. As a means of recording each lesson for parent and therapist, the child is encouraged to bring a large scrapbook to each session. As the therapist works, the programme is written into this book. If it is possible, the schedule can be repeated with mother during the week. Successes and failures noted by her during the week allow the therapist to determine whether therapy goals have been realistic.

The initial interview

The importance of a well structured and detailed history taking is well known. When working with the learning disabled child, particular attention should be paid to the following areas:

Birth history

Family history of learning disability

Intermittent or persistent middle ear disease, especially in infancy and the pre-school years. Conductive hearing loss seems to exacerbate underlying learning disability by preventing the child from attending to, listening to, processing and recalling auditory information which is the basis of language learning

School reports. Negative comments recur term after term

Speech and language skills in the home, the schoolroom and the playground. (Lucas, 1980.) Most children and adolescents with specific learning disability find it difficult to respond appropriately to the use of complex and abstract language. Parents often tell us that their children appear not to listen, that their behaviour is consequently inappropriate. However, they may also report that they talk 'very well'. But many of these children cannot follow a conversation between their parents about the need to conserve energy, how Aunt Anne hurt her leg because she is elderly and arthritic, that Jane's birthday present is a surprise. A visit to a museum becomes remembered for the sweets bought at the gift shop, because the child cannot absorb what he is seeing without simplistic, repetitive, verbal explanation.

Many parents do not realize that the type of language needed in the classroom, or in a museum, is very different from that at the dinner table or playground, and we should help them to become aware of the different patterns of communication required in the diverse situations that make up their child's life. During the first interview, discussion with the parents will highlight the most urgent areas for consideration by the language therapist. A more formal assessment then follows where we assess the understanding, use of, and production of spoken language.

Assessing the understanding of spoken language

(Assessment of this aspect of communication is complex and varied. We should pay particular attention to aspects of the child's understanding of single words and beyond this to his comprehension of complex linguistic structures in a variety of situations.)

RECEPTIVE VOCABULARY

The British Picture Vocabulary Scale (Dunn *et al*, 1982) is a most useful tool for assessing receptive vocabulary at the single word level. Learning disabled children may score at, below, or above age level. We should carefully assess the type of errors made by the child during testing. Some children confuse words which are phonologically similar; others, words which are semantically similar. Some pictures may be visually misidentified. Moreover, it is important to be alert to the possibility that, even though a child might score within the average range for the comprehension of single words, he may still demonstrate a naming difficulty which seriously hampers his expressive skills (Wiig and Becker-Caplan, 1984; Nelson and Warrington, 1980; Luria, 1966).

Clifford is nine years and eight months old. His teacher suspected he was hard of hearing. He did not concentrate and his comprehension skills were poor. He had difficulty understanding the concepts of mathematics. His reading and spelling were below age average. He spelt 'knocker' as 'noker'; 'born' as 'bron'; 'fly' as 'flight'. He read 'ache' as 'ank'; 'bough' as 'bo'; 'quay' as 'kway'; 'sphere' as 'sere'. Although there was a history of slow speech and language develop-ment, his parents did not feel that at the time he was referred for reading therapy he had any 'language difficulty', and a superficial examination did not reveal the extent of his underlying linguistic failures. An audiogram and tympanogram revealed that he suffered from 'glue ear', and probably had done, intermittently, for some years. It is also important to point out that although Clifford had much difficulty with written language, an optometrist found no evidence of eye or muscle preference or weakness, nor of any visual perceptual difficulties. There was a family history of specific learning difficulty. Clifford presented for remedial help when preparing for a major examination, a time when we mostly see children who have moderate learning disabilities.

On the BPVS, Clifford scored at the 28th percentile, which represented a receptive vocabulary age of 8 years and 8 months. (His C.A. it will be recalled, was 9.8 yrs.) During the test he confused several visual stimuli; pointing to 'fish hook' for 'arrow'; 'hammering' for 'chopping'; 'nurse' for 'dentist'; 'feathery' for 'furry'; 'vegetables' for 'fruit'; 'horn' for 'tusk'; 'astronomer' for 'archaeologist'. Possibly, Clifford had visually misidentified the stimuli (Wiig and Becker-Caplan, 1984). However, when he was asked to name a series of picture cards he made the same errors, repeatedly. His performance suggested that he understood the functional relationships between words but he did not possess precise semantic representations of them. (See Table 4.1.)

Luria wrote extensively about the nominative function of language and he has reminded us that 'when we name an object we must select from ... possible alternatives one association, inhibit all the rest ... and carry out an operation analogous to that taking place during differentiation' (1966, p.397).

Picture Stimulus	Verbal Response
rope	string
bear	dog
torch	light, shine, dunno
air-balloon	parachute
lamb	dog
tractor	combinder ... a combinder harvester? ... I know what it look (sic) like
constellation	conclussion (he and his mother had earlier spoken about concussion)

Table 4.1 Naming errors made by Clifford, C. A. 9 years 8 months

During treatment we attempted to direct Clifford's awareness to the semantic markers of words. We used school texts and well illustrated books from the library to highlight some of the functional and compositional attributes of words. If Clifford called a 'slipper' a 'shoe', we looked at pictures of each object, and talked about the differences between the items. We talked about use, texture, smell, colour, sound. As soon as he became more skilful in naming pictures accurately, we reduced his reliance on visual aids, and spoke about the words and how we might classify and categorize them. We have found 'Another World', published by Schofield and Sims, and 'The First Thousand Words', published by Usborne, to be useful workbooks.

Thus it seems that while the learning disabled child is listening to language, his ability to lay down the correct patterns associated with a particular word may be compromised; etiology may be unknown, or may be due to the interaction of numerous neurological and environmental factors (Brainerd, 1982; Johnson, 1980; Kirk, 1983; Lerner, 1981; Valett, 1980; Young, 1978). When a child is asked, under pressure of accuracy and speed, to choose the correct word from a group which are similar in sound, appearance and function, he may not respond accurately. Can he answer correctly in less formal settings, or does a word-retrieval difficulty dog all his endeavours? This is an important factor for the therapist and the parent to observe and remediate.

While it is said that the learning disabled child should be treated by therapists who use the 'multi-sensory' approach (for critical evaluation of this view see Vellutino, 1983; Gaddes, 1980), it might be that we have to teach a boy like Clifford (who has thousands of misrepresented words in his vocabulary) through spoken language at the outset with appropriate illustrations. We hope that by teaching Clifford the *principle* that all objects and ideas have markers with which we can hang them in particular 'closets', he will generalize categories of sounds, words and ideas for himself. We will talk to Clifford about the touch, the smell, the sound, the look of, the movement of a parachute. We cannot hope to produce one in treatment. He must learn to use language in the spoken and then the written form, to develop an appreciation of words and ideas in every area of communication.

COMPLEX VERBAL LINGUISTIC STRUCTURES

It is extremely difficult to assess and remediate the understanding of complex verbal linguistic structures. As many aspects of this function as possible should be examined and therefore items have to be drawn from different tests (Woodcock and Johnson, 1982; Luria, 1966; Wiig and Semel, 1980; Johnson, 1980; Blalock, 1981; Goodglass and Kaplan, 1972; Hammill and Newcomer, 1982; Bishop, 1982). Where a child has difficulty in a certain area, more detailed tests should follow so that specific and appropriate treatment can be planned.

The following are some of the areas which require examination and treatment.

Syntax: plurals, pronouns, passive, genitive, tense

There are several tests which assess how well the child comprehends syntactic structures. The TROG Test of Reception of Grammar (Bishop, 1982) is useful with younger children, while Wiig and Semel's Clinical Evaluation of Language Functions (1980), a test of linguistic structure, memory and semantics, is appropriate as a screening device with older children. The Woodcock–Johnson Psycho-Educational Battery, together with all the tests designed by Hammill and his colleagues (see Test References, p. 78), provide useful information about the school-going child.

To illustrate one of the difficulties which learning disabled children have with many types of linguistic structures, we shall look at the case of Sally, who had difficulty with the comprehension of the passive voice.

Sally is 15 years and 9 months old. She has a verbal I.Q. of 115 and a Performance I.Q. of 125 (WISC-R). She has a history of poor reading and spelling skills; her maternal uncle is 'dyslexic'. Sally's English teacher was concerned about her difficulty in relating verbal information in the correct sequence succinctly, and her consequent problems with creative writing. She scored at the 60th percentile on the BPVS (see below for description of her naming difficulties), and at the superior level on the GAPADOL Reading Comprehension Test. (McCloed, 1973).

Sally was unwilling to answer this question:

The tiger was bitten by the lion. Who was bitten?

She asked the therapist to repeat the structure but was still unable to respond.

During the course of treatment, Sally responded verbally to specific structures in this manner:

The oranges are squozen; the boy was bit by the dog.

She rarely used the passive form in creative writing, and when she did, the same errors (neologisms, reduced forms) were noted as those in oral language.

During treatment, to encourage more fluent use of unusual verb structures, we used pictures taken from magazines, depicting action scenes. We spoke about them in the present, past and future tenses and then we transferred to the passive form, e.g.

The woman is typing a letter. Yesterday she typed a letter. Tomorrow she will type a letter. The letter is being typed by the woman. Yesterday the letter was typed by the woman.

Sally was asked to find six pictures each week, and to tape her responses at home. We then monitored her efforts together the following session. For the third session she was asked to write sentences in the passive form for six new pictures. To make sure she was using the structures correctly, she recorded them, listened to them, and when she was satisfied they were correct, she wrote them down.

It is a repeated observation during treatment that, if oral discussion precedes writing instead of the other way round, the written form is more mature, fluent and stable (Phelps-Gunn, 1982; Hammill and Larsen, 1983). Most syntactic errors may be treated in the manner described above. Naturally age will determine whether one uses real objects for demonstration or illustrations. It is most helpful to use school material wherever possible. If we use the syntactic structures which Sally finds in her text books as therapy tools, she will be able more easily to carry over her skills from treatment to the classroom.

Absurdities, Puns, Proverbs, Quantification

During school years, children use increasingly complicated language operations to move from one-step thinking (the concrete level) to more complex and abstract constructs. (See Piaget, Luria, Menyuk, Bloom, Crystal, among others, for theoretical considerations.) Children with specific learning disability have difficulty tuning into the nuances of spoken language, for example: the meaning of a proverb, idiom, pun, or absurdity. Martin was just such a child.

Martin was 13 years and 6 months old. He presented with a persistent history of reading and writing failure. His hearing and vision were within normal limits. Speech and language development were slow. At the age of six he was seen briefly by a speech therapist for f/th and s/th articulation errors. His *language* function was never assessed. Yet at the age of 13 his auditory processing was obviously below normal limits, his expressive language equally limited. Mother reported that his teachers seemed only concerned with the fact that he could hardly read and spell, that his handwriting was appalling. His verbal I.Q. on the WISC-R was 102 and his score on the BPVS was found to be at the 45th percentile. Martin produced some interesting error patterns throughout the test sequence. Here we see how he responded verbally to the presentation of spoken idioms and proverbs.

Q: *A stitch in time saves nine?*
A: When you have to stitch up something ... you might not have time later.

Q: *She gave the game away?*
A: She lost dreadfully!

Q: *Playing for time?*
A: Playing to make the time go by.

Presenting the same phrases in writing did nothing to help Martin's comprehension of the structure. He remained unable to attribute an abstract meaning to the words. We then used some items which appear in tests designed by Goodglass and Kaplan, Daniels and Dyack and Woodcock and Johnson, and observed that Martin could not answer the following questions correctly.

Do guitars play? . . . . . . Yes.

Are blue jeans red? . . . . . . Yes.

Place the ring above the pencil . . . . . . I don't get it. What must I do?

Martin's comprehension of abstract terminology was limited. Words which appear in scientific texts at school such as: multiples, calculate, estimate, approximate, capacity, denominator, depth, equivalent, symmetry, pair, share – all seemed to be beyond his comprehension. Comparative linguistic forms such as 'heavier than', 'farther than' proved difficult (Wiig and Semel, 1980). If these and other similar terms occurred in the text, he could not solve the problem. These difficulties are not simply related to his inability to read some of the words, for when we discussed them verbally in different contexts to elicit comprehension, Martin still could not understand their use. His difficulties were further complicated by the fact that he found it hard to follow a verbal sequence where he had to determine how certain chemical, physical or mathematical reactions occurred.

It seemed important to try to assess why these incorrect responses were occurring. Martin was unable to respond to the linguistic complexity of the sentence. It is well known that embedding within a short sentence may cause more errors than a longer, simpler sentence will do. On the other hand, length of utterance may hamper response, rather than the type of linguistic structure contained therein, so careful analysis of error patterns is important.

Martin only resolved his difficulties in Mathematics when concrete examples of size, shape and quantity were demonstrated, and only gradually could more abstract concepts be introduced. Definition of terms in the text were stressed, and the dictionary became as valuable a tool as the calculator. (See below for Martin's naming difficulties.) Where the structure of the sentence proved problematic we wrote each word on a separate index card in different colours. Martin tried to restructure the sentence correctly. He tried to substitute words which might lead to the same meaning. We tried to learn about the deep and surface structure of sentences in the spoken and written form. A very useful series of Mathematics workbooks proved to be the PSM Series (Stagg, 1984), which although designed for children who do not have learning disabilities, have such excellent illustrations and verbal explanations that Martin was able to follow the mathematical principles very easily.

Analogies

In order to understand the analogy 'spider is to fly, as cat is to mouse', a child must be able to process several linguistic concepts simultaneously. The solution of structures like analogies requires the child to '... perceive and abstract an expressed semantic relationship between two words and use that relationship in a second context' (Wiig and Semel, 1980, p. 210). Some learning disabled children seem unable to use verbal thinking skills in a sophisticated, two-step manner, and therefore find this task difficult. Their responses are complicated by poor general knowledge, poor learning strategies and limited vocabulary.

Simon was 13 years and 8 months old. He began to talk when he was three and a half. He had suffered two epileptic seizures following a high fever at 6 months. No neurological signs were present on further examination but he displayed unusual behavioural patterns. He was labelled as 'very disturbed' by the educational authorities when he made little progress at his local school, and was taken into analytic treatment for two years at the age of eight. His communication skills, and consequently his ability to relate to people, were poor but Simon was *never* assessed by a language therapist. At the age of ten his parents were advised by psychologists to put him into a school for maladjusted children. However they were fortunate to meet a reading therapist who recognized not only that Simon had severe reading and writing problems, but that he also had a severe receptive and expressive language disorder.

Today Simon attends an excellent comprehensive school, where he is a member of the rugby team and achieves average grades in all subjects, except Mathematics. His teachers and friends definitely do not regard him as maladjusted or disturbed. His verbal skills remain limited, and he takes a long time to process complex, abstract instructions. He finds auditory processing alone very difficult, and must have visual stimuli to clarify the issue at hand. He and Martin are similar in many respects and his responses to a task of analogies revealed some of his deficiencies.

Spider is to fly, as cat is to ... dog.

Sheep is to mutton, as pig is to ... beef.

Uncle is to ... mother .., as aunt is to niece.

Artist is to ... paint .., as author is to book.

Simon indicated that he was able to think of the correct categories: animals, relatives, etc, but he had been unable to carry his verbal thinking skills one step further, to deduce that spiders and cats are predators, a fly is a victim, therefore the answer must be 'bird' or 'mouse'. He understood that he was to produce a sub-category of the group 'meat', but could only retrieve a word which was semantically related to the target word. At times he produced the incorrect part of speech – a verb (paint), where a noun (painting) was appropriate.

An analysis of errors in this manner indicated how treatment might proceed. In addition to his other language difficulties, Simon needed specific help with parts of speech, classification and categorization of words, and learning to use words logically to solve problems. While Simon, Martin and Sally all revealed many obstacles in the quest for the understanding of verbal language, they also had difficulty producing spoken language.

Assessing the Child's Production of Spoken Language

The use of language for conversation, creative writing and academic proficiency may be restricted for the learning disabled by many of the factors discussed above. Poor word retrieval, poor understanding of abstract concepts and deficits in verbal short and long term memory, all merge to contribute to limited conversation, immature written work and lack of participation in the classroom (Wiig and Semel, 1980; Phelps–Gunn and Phelps–Terasaki, 1982; Wren, 1983).

Confrontation naming

Many studies have reported the relationship between specific learning disability, restricted language performance and naming disorders (Nelson and Warrington, 1980; German, 1982; Wiig and Becker–Caplan, 1984). From a practical point of view, the majority of children (of varying ages) who are referred for *language* therapy after psychologial assessment for reading difficulties present with a word-finding difficulty. The word-retrieval problem may be most evident in picture naming, but it can also be observed in sentence completion tasks and in activities which involve semantic categorization.

Sean was a boy who presented with marked word-finding difficulties. He was seven years old and had a full scale I.Q. of 107. During the course of treatment he produced errors of several types including circumlocutions (for 'spade' he said 'use it for the mud'), imprecise responses (for 'dentist' he said 'toothman'; for 'shoulder' he said 'ball and socket'), and semantic paraphasias (for 'heel' he said 'elbow'; 'hose' for 'tap', and 'nose' for 'beak').

A second child, Linda, was eleven when she presented with poor comprehension, reduced verbal I.Q., but with a performance score that was high average. She had experienced early reading and spelling difficulties and now her teacher was concerned about poor maths skills and an inability to concentrate in the classroom. Examples of her naming errors are shown in Table 4.2.

Target Word	Response
smoke	fire
tube	I don't know
fountain	waterfall
arch	oval
chain	ring
crayfish	eel
hatching	becoming alive
wing	feather

Table 4.2 Errors made by Linda, aged 11, on a picture-naming task

Linda's incorrect responses remained constant from one session to the next, suggesting she had only a passive understanding of word meanings. In therapy we worked on the similarities and differences between words and tried to develop effective word-retrieval strategies. We concentrated on games like Pelmanism, word association, guessing the categories of words which started with a particular sound, and so on. Her word flexibility improved slowly, allowing her to communicate more meaningfully.

It goes without saying that if a word retrieval difficulty reflects inadequate word knowledge, as it seemed to in Linda's case, there will be concomitant comprehension difficulties. Lucy at the age of 13 years and 9 months was reported to have poor comprehension in the classroom, as well as early reading and spelling difficulties. Despite such problems, Lucy scored at the 60th percentile on the BPVS. However, her naming difficulties seemed to reflect 'remote, but semantic realizations'. Her responses to other tests in this series (e.g. idioms, analogies) showed limited ability to use language creatively, with a restricted, concrete use of words. A good example of her comprehension difficulties emerged during a discussion about Egyptology, which she was studying at school:

Lucy was asked: *What is the name for an Egyptian tomb?*

She replied: A mummy.

She was asked: *What is a mummy?*

Lucy replied: Where females were put when they died.

Another example shows that there was, for her, only one application for the word 'smell', and she spoke of:

... the smell of perfume ...

We found we could describe 'smells' in different ways: body odour ... essence of vanilla ... fumes of petrol ... scent of perfume ... smell of cooking ... and so on. We put the words into sentences, to build graphic word-pictures. To expand her expressive vocabulary we worked on the classification and categorization of words. Children like Lucy are often described as having poor verbal fluency. If we ask them to list the 'members' of the 'family' *TRANSPORT*, they may not be able to make the division into rail, sea, air and land spontaneously. Further breakdown of those categories into their constituent members also proves very difficult. In time, with specific tuition, the idea of using words creatively and in differing contexts does become a basic principle and generalization takes over from our detailed explanations of how and why words belong to different groups.

Repetition of words and phrases

Numerous tests are available for determining the accuracy of recall of words and phrases of increasing length and complexity (Wiig and Semel, 1980; Goodglass and Kaplan, 1972). Martin, aged 13 years and 6 months, had difficulty coping with syntactic and/or semantic complexity, as opposed to length of utterance. Although his articulation was perfect in spontaneous speech, articulation errors were evident in his reproduction of low probability sentences. For example:

Wasn't the rhinoceros crossed by the river ... became ...
Was the ricono crossed the river ...

The phantom soared across the foggy heath ... became ...
The santin soared across the soggy feat.

The spy fled to Greece ... became ...
The spear thread Greek.

Similarly, there may be difficulties with the repetition of single words, especially those which are multisyllabic. For example, Sean, aged seven, mispronounced the following words:

Hospital... became... hotipal; *speech therapy*... speak through; *hippopotamus*... hittotamus; *emerald*... enemald; *distribution*... distribrution ...

Children with the above difficulties will be particularly at risk in the classroom when exposed to unfamiliar words and phrases. Since they cannot automatically reproduce such information, they will have great difficulty recalling new material.

Sean's teacher was very concerned that he could not follow instructions given to the class as a whole and in particular was unable to begin a task or lay it out correctly, until she was able to supervise him individually. We realized that he could only retain three instructions at a time, and fewer if complex linguistic structures were embedded in the sequence. His poor receptive vocabulary prevented him from understanding many of the words contained within written and verbal instructions. His teacher kept a careful record of these for a week and was then able to report to the therapist and the parents exactly what his difficulties were. In short, many learning disabled children have limited verbal short-term memory, their sequencing skills are poor and their receptive vocabulary is reduced. The teacher needs information from the therapist about how she might treat such a child if he is not to fall behind with his work, especially that of a complex nature. Sentences in therapy have to be carefully controlled and graded. The therapist must ensure whether she needs to control for length and/or complexity of utterance, for parts of speech and vocabulary, and memory skills should also be heightened within this framework (see Piaget, Baddeley, Wilson, Pressly, Wiig and Semel, Wren, Johnson and Myklebust).

Conversation, story-telling and verbal description

The above examples illustrate that it can be difficult for the learning disabled child to communicate in a free-flowing, creative and interesting manner. Parents and teachers sometimes describe these children as shy or withdrawn, although often these are the children who are searching for the right word, who circumlocute – who generally seem to have symptoms of the expressive language difficulties outlined above. On the other hand, there are learning disabled children who chatter endlessly, but their language may be empty and repetitive.

It is important to assess how the learning disabled child responds to tasks designed to elicit a free flow of language, especially if under pressure. Goodglass and Kaplan (1972, p.25) used a black and white line drawing to assess conversational speech in dysphasic subjects and observed that 'The vocabulary constraints of the picture bring out the word-finding difficulty more sharply.'

In an informal manner a child can be presented with a suitable colour picture (perhaps one taken from a Sunday Colour Supplement) and asked to look carefully at it and to describe what he sees. In addition, he should be asked to say what he thinks happened *before* the picture was taken, and what might happen *next*. He can then be asked to make up an imaginary story about a second picture, and to give it a title.

Clifford was presented with a picture of a village green, where people were playing cricket, strolling, and so on. This was his response:

'Dark green grass. The house beside it. Ten foot long. Runs. Rain. Bowling person'.

He could not develop this very sparse description and certainly was unable to consider what might have taken place before or afterwards. He became quite sullen during this task – a response which is not uncommon, so great is the stress when speech is demanded in a propositional task. The learning disabled child usually responds more easily to a series of picture sequences where the story progression is visually evident (John Horniman Story Pack, 1972).

Martin's response to the dog chasing the cat story sequence was as follows:

'... all sudden the dog ran away. It had such a good strongth. The cat, her hairs stuck up like as a magnet above her. She ran up a tree.'

It is useful to use picture card series with the more severely disabled child as a starting point to improve the flexibility and elaboration of expressive language. Provided that the child can sequence the cards, he should be encouraged to describe exactly what he sees in the first card, and so on to the last. Observations may be recorded on to tape, and altered, if the child wishes. The particular sequence of the story can then be discussed, and this should also be recorded. At first children may dislike recording their observations but, with encouragement, they gradually become more fluent. This activity can be enlarged upon by creating alternative stories for the same pictures, or making up new, imaginary stories. When the children are more adept at verbal skills the stories can be transferred to the written form. In the first instance they can be encouraged to use their tapes as if they were dictaphones, as this technique helps written fluency to improve steadily.

Another useful tool for improving expressive language skill is to ask the child to describe accurately how they might go about their favourite activity (fishing, baking a cake, putting together a model car). The specific verbal sequences required for such tasks are not easily retrievable at first, so picture series may again be useful. In addition, the excellent books published by Ladybird, MacDonald, and Usborne, among others, may be constructively used by parents and therapists. Many parents seem reluctant to read non-fiction books to their children. They often ask: 'Where can I buy that book, it looks so interesting, but I never see them around!' To help the willing parent, the therapist should explore the local book and toy libraries so she can direct him or her in the right direction and show how easily the child's word power can be increased by using books which have been especially designed for that purpose.

Memory and Sequencing

Few would dispute that short-term and long-term memory processes underlie language behaviour, and there is considerable evidence that children with specific learning difficulties are subject to a variety of *verbal* memory deficits (see Rack and Snowling, this volume). If the sequences which have been memorized since infancy are considered, it is interesting to note how many learning disabled children have failed to retain nursery rhymes, days of the week, months of the year, rules of games, rules of the home, and so on.

These are aspects of spoken language which are repeated over and over in many different contexts and yet still they create difficulty. The older the child, the more sophisticated his skills of recall need be because he will need to memorize not only automatic sequences of the type mentioned, but also intricate details of the spoken and written words presented by his teacher and textbooks. This section outlines some of the most frequent problems encountered by learning disabled children and, by reference to specific cases, suggests ways in which they might be managed.

1) *Months and days*

Teaching Clifford to remember the names of the months of the year proved to be an exacting task. He could not recall them by auditory emphasis alone, so we found a large board of card. On the left hand side we wrote the months. The four seasons were represented by four appropriate colours. In the next column, in different colours, we wrote how many days there are in each month. The next column was devoted to illustrating special occasions which occurred during particular months.

The board was hung next to Clifford's bed, so he could recite them each evening. At the same time his mother would ask: What month is it? What day is it today? What was yesterday? What day will it be tomorrow?

This allowed him to improve his understanding of the order of the days – a concept about which he was still uncertain at the beginning of treatment.

2) *Rules of the game*

Sean could not play soccer because of his inability to listen to, and retain, a *sequence* of verbal information. He had no visuo-spatial difficulties, so when his mother sat with him, discussed the rules, and illustrated the sequence of play, his game improved. His sports master also monitored Sean more carefully, to ensure he executed a new sequence correctly.

This example serves to illustrate that adequate *comprehension* of the task to be remembered is essential. Children with specific learning disability may need to have new concepts explained *practically*, and perhaps *visually*, before they can approach a level where they need fewer clues to arrive at the correct solution. We have to use many different words to explain the same idea to them. Even when a new concept is understood, it may have to be rehearsed daily for learning to be effective.

3) *Learning tables*

Many children with specific learning difficulties have a good concept of number but find arithmetic problematic. Very many cannot learn their tables; Martin was just such a child. At the age of thirteen and a half, he had reached a stage where it was vital for him to be able to manipulate numbers in his mind if his performance in mathematics was not to be jeopardized.

We wrote out the tables on index cards as shown in Figure 4.1:

Each number and symbol was written in a different colour.

We also put the table to be learned onto tape:

Once nine is ...... (silent gap) .... nine, and so on.

Martin listened to the tape as he looked at the appropriate cards. During the silent gap in the tape he had to supply the correct answer, which immediately followed the silence and, by reversing the card he was holding, he was able to see the correct answer. Children who are able to understand the concept of the tables do learn quickly by this method. Where they fail, one has to return to concrete operations, and teaching may be prolonged.

4) *Learning for tests*

At one time or another the learning disabled child has to study school material for tests. Retaining the information is very difficult. The children often do not know how to organize themselves sufficiently, where to begin, nor what strategies might be useful to help them to learn the necessary material efficiently and permanently. At first, parents may have to be closely involved in helping their children plan study schedules, how to make sense of texts, what information should be retained, and what discarded.

To illustrate the difficulties which the learning disabled child may face, some of the elements of a history syllabus will be examined. History is a subject which most children learn. It is therefore surprising to see the difficulty of the texts with which they must cope, and the details they are expected to remember. Many textbooks may fail to take into account the linguistic competence of the reader, so parents of children with specific learning disabilities should be encouraged to elaborate upon the topics introduced at school using suitable supplementary non-fiction books from their local library, taking care to look

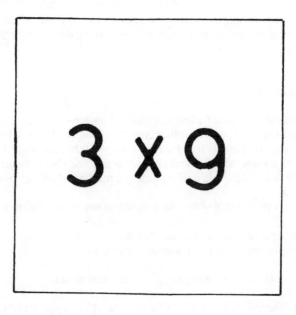

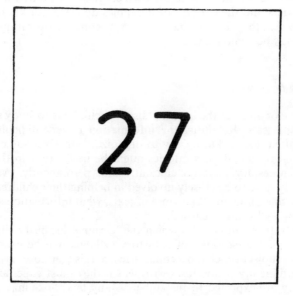

Figure 4.1 Illustration of cards used for teaching tables in a multisensory manner. (Front and reverse sides shown)

for simplified texts and interesting illustrations. An excellent series is MacDonald's 'Peoples of the Past'. Figure 2 illustrates a paragraph from one of the books, 'The Romans', by Joan Forman.

Gladiators

A more terrible form of 'entertainment' took place in the amphitheatre. It was here that gladiators, or men and wild animals, fought to the death in front of large audiences. Criminals, prisoners, and later, Christians, were put into the arena to face lions and tigers that had been kept hungry for the occasion.

These displays were the favourite shows of the Roman people for several centuries. The mob in the amphitheatre had no pity for a wounded gladiator. If he was wounded in a fight, he was killed. A wounded gladiator was not thought to be of any use to anyone.

The largest amphitheatre in the Roman World was the Colosseum. The opening of the Colosseum in AD 80 was celebrated with a hundred days of continuous games.

Figure 4.2 An extract from 'The Romans' by Joan Forman. MacDonald. (p.30)[1]

Details might be learnt in the following way:

Let's think of other words for: terrible, fight, audiences, hungry, display, century.

What do you think an amphitheatre looked like?

Look at this picture of the gladiator. Describe everything you see in this picture. Move from the top of the picture and work right through it. Try to notice every detail.

What action words can you find in the passage? Let's make sentences with each of them.

Now tell me in your own words about 'Gladiators'.

Let's put that onto tape. Listen to what you have said. Does it match what you have read in the passage? Let's check.

Now write down the 'Key Words' from this passage on separate cards, in different colours. We will write down the most important words which tell us the most about 'Gladiators'.

Tomorrow, take out your cards, and look at them. Listen to your tape, and read the passage again. Ask Mum to work with you, and see how much of the passage you can remember. Tell her all about 'Gladiators'. You should try to talk about what you have learned each day until the test, so that you won't forget the important details.

[1] This extract is reproduced with the kind permission of the publishers.

In general, provided that information is presented in a structured, systematic and well-categorized manner, the child with a specific learning difficulty will be able to retain it. Without structure the child may be 'at sea'.

Conclusions

A number of writers have commented on the many similarities between learning-disabled child and adult dysphasic patients (Benson and Geschwind, 1969; Denckla and Rudel, 1976; Aaron *et al*, 1980). This view may be useful to the language therapist who has worked with neurologically impaired patients. However, it is important to remember that the language-impaired, learning-disabled child is very different from an adult whose premorbid system was completely intact (Lebrun, 'Personal Communication', 1984). The similarities indicate that effective language assessment procedures, whether designed for children or adults, are all tapping the fundamental structure of a language system which is deficient, for reasons still unspecified.

The assessment and remediation of the learning-disabled child who has associated language difficulties is rewarding and fascinating as each session provides more clues about a particular child's strategies, strengths and weaknesses. Where language therapy is coupled with reading and writing intervention the child can progress rapidly, especially if parents actively share in the treatment process. The therapist requires a flexible and creative attitude toward specific learning disabilities. Although many research questions remain to be answered, it is still possible to assess patients and to set up a management programme attuned to their individual educational and language needs.

Acknowledgements

The writer would like to express her gratitude to Mrs Mary Lobascher, the Principal Clinical Psychologist, The Hospital for Sick Children, Great Ormond Street, London, for her support and encouragement; to Dr Doris J. Johnson, Program Head, Program in Learning Disabilities, Northwestern University, Evanston, Illinois and Avril Klaff, Doctoral Candidate at the same centre, for sharing their expertise in the field of learning disabilities.

Test Material

Bishop, D. (1982). *The TROG Test of Reception of Grammar*.
Disimondi, F. *The Token Test for Children*. Hingham: Teaching Resources.

Dunn, L. M., Dunn, L. M. *et al* (1982). *The British Picture Vocabulary Scale*. Windsor: NFER-NELSON.

Gardiner, M. F. *Expressive One-Word Picture Vocabulary Test*. Novato: Academic Therapy Publications.

Goodglass, H. and Kaplan, E. (1972). *The Assessment of Aphasia and Related Disorders*. Philadelphia: Lea and Febiger.

Hammill, D. D., Brown, V. L., *et al* (1980). *TOAL – Test of Adolescent Language*. Austen: Pro-ed.

Hammill, D. D., and Larsen, S. C. (1983). *TOWL – The Test of Written Language*. Austin: Pro-ed.

John Horniman Staff with Marian Bunzl (1973). *Story Pack*. London: JCAA Publications.

McCloed, J. and Anderson, J. (1973). *GAP and GAPADOL Reading Comprehension*. London: Heinemann Educational.

Semel, E. M. and Wiig, E. H. (1980). *Clinical Evaluation of Language Function – CELF*. Columbus: Charles E. Merrill.

Woodcock, R. W. and Johnson, M. B. (1982). *Woodcock–Johnson Psycho-Educational Battery*. Hingham: Teaching Resources.

Margaret Snowling

5 The Assessment of Reading and Spelling Skills

In a highly literate society, it is crucial that a child learns to read and spell. To do so is no small achievement, for two complex skills which are both independent and interrelated have to be mastered. It is fortunate that the majority of children become proficient users of written language with only the minimum of supervision. Unfortunately, there remain a significant proportion who encounter specific difficulty. Before discussing ways of assessing the teaching needs of these children, it is important for us to consider what constitutes normal reading and spelling development, and this will provide a framework within which we can consider both various aspects of reading disorder and individual differences in reading and spelling skill.

Reading and Spelling: Similarities and Differences

Traditionally, reading and spelling have been considered two inter-related processes with the latter 'parasitic' upon the former. Spelling has received relatively little attention in its own right, although it has been recognized for some time that brain damage can selectively impair an individual's ability to read without affecting spelling (as in cases of alexia without agraphia). Most recently, it has become accepted that reading and spelling are different processes (Shallice, 1981; Beauvois and Derouesne, 1979), with the distinction being most clearly visible in the early stages (Frith, 1985). For example, Bryant and Bradley (1980) showed that beginning readers can often spell words which they cannot read. Their subjects could most easily read visually distinctive, irregular words such as 'school', 'light' and 'biscuit', while they could most easily spell short, regular words such as 'bun', 'sit' and 'frog'. On these grounds, Bryant and Bradley argued that early reading is visually based and early spelling is dependent upon sound.

More generally, Frith and Frith (1980) have argued that an important difference between reading and spelling is that reading is a recognition process while spelling is a retrieval process. Thus, reading can proceed using 'partial cues'. Indeed this is why techniques such as speed reading which require only minimum visual analysis of words can work. In contrast, spelling requires the use of full cues. To spell

80

well, words must be represented in a detailed way in the mind of a speller and this memory image must be recoverable. In the absence of spelling knowledge, an individual will be forced to spell words according to the way they sound (Ellis, 1982). They will adopt a 'spell by ear' strategy (Frith, 1979). In the English orthography, reliance on a sound strategy is unsatisfactory and, because of the many seemingly 'arbitrary' conventions, phonetic spelling errors occur (e.g. mewsishun, coppies, percieve).

In short, reading relies on visual processes, spelling upon phonological (sound) processes. To this extent they are independent of each other. However, it is important to note that in order to possess full cues for spelling, detailed analysis of printed words is necessary. The normal reader may carry this out spontaneously during reading or else through the examination of words outside of the context of reading. To the extent that accurate spelling relies upon information derived through reading, spelling is dependent upon it. For this reason, any theory concerning the development of written language skill must account not only for the independence of spelling and reading, but also for the *dependence* of spelling upon reading.

The Development of Reading and Spelling

Frith (1985) describes the child as passing through three phases during the acquisition of literacy: the logographic, the alphabetic and the orthographic. Transition through the phases does not move along simultaneously for reading and spelling.

Reading during the logographic phase is based upon crude 'visual' features. Visually similar words are likely to be confused, e.g. 'lorry' and 'yellow' because they both contain 'l' and 'y'. At this stage the child is not aware of the importance of letter order in printed words. Marsh *et al* (1980) argued that visual reading is not conducive to good spelling, and indeed, spelling at this stage is minimal – a child may only be willing to write one or two highly familiar words (perhaps their own name and some everyday words).

The alphabetic phase is entered first for spelling and subsequently it seems that these skills are transferred to reading. What happens is that children wishing to write have only impoverished images of printed words; therefore, they start to spell words as they sound. Early spelling attempts, such as those documented by Bissex (1980) in her book 'GNYS at work' (genius at work), demonstrate well this reliance upon sound. However, before a child is able to understand the relationships between letters and sounds embodied in printed words, it is necessary for a state of 'phoneme awareness' to have been reached. For this reason, a child must understand that spoken words can be segmented into phonemes. This is no mean achievement for a child. Liberman and Shankweiler (1979) suggested that the ability to do so is seldom apparent prior to the age of 6 and there is ample evidence that acquisition of this knowledge presents a stumbling block for many children (Rozin and Gleitman, 1977).

Provided a child *can* make this conceptual advance, it is possible to go on to perfect alphabetic skills, particularly through spelling (Snowling and Perin, 1983), and moreover, having entered the alphabetic phase for spelling, most children soon attempt to transfer their new strategy to the reading situation. This move will allow them to tackle new words which they have never seen before and to develop proficient 'word attack' skills.

It follows that there are some important distinctions between the logographic and the alphabetic phases. Firstly, a child with logo-graphic skills can read only familiar words, while the child in the alphabetic phase can make use of a system of letter–sound relation-ships to decipher unfamiliar words, such as nonwords. Secondly, spelling in the logographic phase is minimal but in the alphabetic phase it can (at least) be phonetic.

Thirdly and finally, the child enters the orthographic phase, which is really the phase which characterizes adult literacy. Now the child has access to abstract representations of printed words. These allow accurate reading and automatic spelling. It is possible that the detailed representations are the result of an amalgamation of logographic and alphabetic strategies. Words may have first been registered in a global manner in an internal lexicon during the logographic phase. During the alphabetic phase, the use of letter–sound rules during reading redirects attention to the internal left to right structure of printed words. The orthographic information which this analysis exposes may be written into the already existing lexical representation, for subsequent use during the orthographic phase. During the orthographic phase, reading and writing are both analytic, but independent of sound.

Learning to read and spell: task demands and 'at risk' factors

Frith's (1985) theory of reading and spelling development makes clear that the acquisition process will make different demands at different points in time. At each 'critical' stage the child must bring specialized resources to the learning situation if written language development is to proceed normally. If children do not, for whatever reason, have access to these resources, they will be at risk of failing, that is, unable to progress to the next phase.

It seems likely that, during the logographic phase, children rely almost entirely upon those skills which are utilized in everyday life for memorizing other visual events. Just as children learn the names for pictures, they will, with only a little more sophistication, acquire a sight vocabulary. Of course to do this children must be exposed to print, they must be motivated to learn and they must be able to attend selectively. They also must be free from perceptual problems and able to integrate visual and verbal information. These are the skills we expect of our four- and five-year-old children who are entering school. Children with specific learning difficulties, who are bright and perceptive, do not usually encounter 'failure' at this stage. However, there can un-doubtedly be problems for the child with difficulties with attention control, memory function or word finding. Fortunately, in all but a minority, the initial slowness can be resolved and logographic skills will be achieved. Although it is not central to this chapter, it is more likely to be children with extreme language delay and/or mental retardation who have trouble in acquiring logographic skills.

It has already been argued that, in order for a child to enter the alphabetic phase, phoneme awareness is necessary. But this is not the only requirement. In order to spell alphabetically, the child needs to be able to segment the sound stream and to memorize and sequence sound segments. To be able to transfer alphabetic knowledge to the reading situation, the child must know of letter–sound relationships and be able to blend or assemble sound segments to synthesize whole words. Since alphabetic competence makes demands upon various aspects of auditory and phonological processing, many children with a history of speech and language problems have difficulty in mastering the alphabetic principle. Recent evidence indicates that children with persisting speech problems and phonological disorder are particularly 'at risk' (see Stackhouse, this volume). Moreover, Frith (1985) has argued convincingly that classic developmental dyslexia reflects a failure to break through to the alphabetic phase. Dyslexic children typically retain logographic skills as shown by the high preponderance of visual errors in their reading attempts:

'instruction' for 'institution'

'champagne' for 'campaign'

'biography' for 'bibliography'

and the nonphonetic nature of their spelling errors:

'anofe' for 'enough'

'tamy' for 'sometimes'

'ac craroo' for 'aquarium'.

Furthermore, there is considerable evidence that dyslexic children have specific difficulty when required to read unfamiliar words out of context. Their nonword reading is typically much poorer than would be expected, given their expertise with real words (Snowling, 1980, 1981; Jorm, 1979; Baddeley, Lewis, Ellis and Miles, 1983).

Thus, the skills required to pass into the alphabetic phase include phoneme awareness, sound segmentation, auditory sequencing, phono-logical memory and phonological assembly. Children with specific learning difficulties display a variety of deficiencies in these processes (Vellutino, 1979) and need specific assistance to facilitate transfer into the alphabetic phase.

Now, if it is true that transition into the orthographic phase is brought about by an amalgamation of logographic and alphabetic strategies, the skills required are specific to written language and derived through experience with this medium. A dyslexic child who has to rely upon sophisticated logographic strategies for reading because alphabetic skills are poor (Temple and Marshall, 1983) will always be somewhat inaccurate in reading, especially when under stress. At best, spelling will be phonetically accurate, but it will be prone to deterioration when full attention cannot be given.

Lastly, there does exist a group of children who are characterized by failure only within the orthographic phase. These children frequently go unrecognized because they have specific spelling difficulties in the absence of reading problems (Frith, 1980). Often they have good use of language with Verbal I.Q. in advance of performance abilities (Naidoo, 1972; Nelson and Warrington, 1974) and they are often reported to have been early readers. It is likely that these children read quickly and fluently, relying heavily upon context, and therefore do not pay close visual attention to the letter by letter structure of words. Consequently, they do not build up detailed lexical representations of words for use in spelling. Their spelling errors are primarily phonetic because alphabetic skills are intact and they have no difficulty in spelling 'by ear'. Speech therapists are less likely to be involved with children of this type although their specifically 'dysgraphic' problems certainly deserve the attention of teachers in any educational setting.

Standardized tests are primarily used to compare the abilities of an individual with those of his or her peers. The value of this procedure is limited, although often important for screening purposes. In clinical work, standardized tests are most important as a means of ascertaining whether achievement in one particular domain (e.g. vocabulary, reading, or arithmetic) is out of line with expectation. For instance, in the normal population, there is substantial correlation between mental age and reading age as determined by standardized tests. 'Bright' children usually read in advance of chronological age whereas 'slow learners' can be expected to be behind the age norm. Epidemiological studies in which the intellectual and scholastic abilities of populations of children are tested permit an unbiased estimate of this correlation. Moreover it is possible by statistical means to derive a regression equation which allows one to predict the level of attainment to be expected of any child in that particular population, given their age and intellectual ability (Yule, 1967).

Perhaps the most recent regression equations available come from the lead studies carried out in London (Yule, Lansdown and Urbana-vicz, 1982). These are shown in Table 5.1. To exemplify their use: a child in London aged 10 years can be expected to have a Reading Age of 10 years 10 months if of above average ability, a Reading Age of 9 years 10 months if of average ability and a Reading Age of 8 years 6 months if mildly retarded. Spelling Ages can be predicted in similar fashion (Table 5.2).

Neale Accuracy $= (-38.86) + (0.63 \times$ FS I.Q.$) + (0.78 \times$ Age$)$
Vernon Spelling $= 25.66 + (0.59 \times$ FS I.Q.$) + (0.11 \times$ Age$)$

Table 5.1 Regression equation based on a primary school population for ages 6–12 years (Yule *et al*, 1982)

C.A.	8 years			9 years			10 years		
I.Q.	80	100	120	80	100	120	80	100	120
R.A. (Neale)	7:02	8:03	9:04	8:00	9:00	10:01	8:09	9:10	10:10
S.A. (Vernon)	6:11	7:11	8:11	7:01	8:00	9:00	7:02	8:02	9:02

Table 5.2 Predicted Reading Ages (Neale Analysis of Reading Ability; Accuracy score) and Spelling Ages (Vernon Test) in a primary school population

In most cases, if reading and spelling ages are in line with expectation, development will be proceeding normally. When either reading or spelling are out of line with expectation, a child can be considered as having a specific learning disability.

Many speech therapists and teachers already make use of the Aston Index (Newton and Thomson, 1976) which outlines a means of testing general ability, against which to examine reading and spelling attainment. There are, of course, many other ways of determining an individual's underlying ability, even if an I.Q. score is not available. The British Picture Vocabulary Scale and Raven's Matrices provide reasonable estimates of verbal and nonverbal abilities and there are a plethora of reading and spelling tests. A comprehensive assessment should include a test of single word reading (favourites are the Schonell Graded Word Reading Test and the Burt (Rearranged) Reading Test) and a test of prose reading (the most extensively used being the Neale Analysis of Reading Ability). When testing spelling, either the Schonell Graded Word Spelling Test or the Vernon Spelling Test can be used. As a quick rule of thumb, Reading Age should be approximately in line with Mental Age, and Spelling Age no more than a year behind reading ability. Any child for whom this is not the case has special educational needs which should be met if considerable underachievement and accompanying psychosocial problems are to be avoided.

It follows that standardized tests of reading and spelling are important for screening purposes and for the detection of specific learning difficulties. One shortcoming of these tests is that they give less information about the stage of reading or spelling acquisition which a child has reached than a teacher or therapist might need. Careful observation during the testing session may suggest which strategies are being used, but if standardized tests are supplemented by a small number of nonstandard procedures, their diagnostic power can be increased significantly. For purposes of qualitative assessment, reading and spelling should be treated separately, always remembering that one process will feed into another. In short, the reading and spelling strategies which an individual habitually adopts must be identified and areas of strength and weakness noted. This will constitute the first step towards a remedial teaching approach attuned to the individual's specific educational needs.

Assessment of Reading Strategies

To describe clearly the means of assessing an individual's reading strategy, it is useful to adopt an information-processing model of the reading process. Although it is difficult to portray the developmental nature of the reading process and the status of the rapidly expanding lexicon, Figure 5.1 serves as a working model. The first strategy which a child adopts (within the logographic phase) is a direct, visually based approach, depicted by route A. Print (written language) is pronounced directly following whole-word recognition and the meanings of words are accessed through links to the semantic memory system (B) which houses the child's knowledge of spoken words (compare a 'look–say' approach).

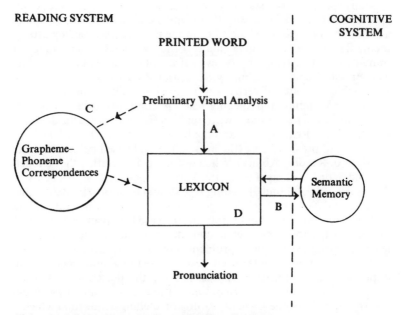

Figure 5.1 Information processing model of reading process

At a somewhat later stage (within the alphabetic phase), a child can adopt a sound approach to words, utilizing knowledge of grapheme–phoneme rules, depicted by route C (compare a phonics approach). The child now has 'visual' and 'phonological' reading strategies available and again, meaning can be addressed. As time progresses, entries in the lexicon become more highly specified (D). These newly acquired and detailed representations of words allow accurate reading and spelling (the orthographic phase). Previous strategies remain accessible in certain circumstances and will be useful, for example, for dealing with unfamiliar words, real names and nonsense words.

It should be noted that the reading system has direct links with the semantic and cognitive systems. These connections account for the fact that we can understand what we read and make predictions about words coming up according to contextual cues (Goodman, 1973). In short, we can bring our general knowledge of the world to bear upon the reading situation. Children with language delay, limited vocabulary or who are of low verbal intelligence will be at risk as far as difficulties with reading comprehension are concerned (see Klein, this volume). However, in most cases of specific learning disability, reading comprehension is constrained only by deficits at the decoding level (Perfetti and Hogaboam, 1975; Stanovich, 1980). If a dyslexic child is presented with reading material at the appropriate reading level, then there is no reason to anticipate conceptual difficulties (Frith and Snowling, 1983). But if, in order to cope with reading material commensurate with intellectual level, an inordinate amount of attention has to be directed towards deciphering the text, then comprehension problems will ensue. It is important for all teachers to be aware of this possibility and to arrange for concessions to be made so that children with specific reading difficulties are not penalized on account of their slow rate of reading, which is often accompanied by inaccuracy. The testing of reading comprehension is a complex and specialized area. Space does not permit detailed discussion as it is the remit of this chapter to discuss those strategies which allow print to be pronounced and to suggest nonstandard procedures for identifying visual and phonological reading skills.

Assessing the balance of visual and phonological skill

Two different observations can provide converging evidence as to whether an individual prefers to adopt a visual or a phonological approach to print. Initially, when presented with a series of single words out of context, the *reading* approach can be observed. Boder (1973) suggests that words read with immediacy form part of a child's sight vocabulary (and therefore are recognized directly) (route A, Figure 5.1). It is then suggested that up to 15 seconds be allowed for the child to apply word-attack processes. (This provides an evaluation of phonological skill – route C, Figure 5.1.) Boder (*ibid*) describes two sorts of pattern. Firstly, a 'dysphonetic' one in which there is a good sight vocabulary but poor word-attack skill. Often 'dyslexic' children either 'know' a word or else they have few strategies available for deciphering it. Boder estimates that around 60 per cent of dyslexics show this pattern. Our clinical experience suggests that children with a history of speech difficulties are especially likely to do so.

A second pattern, shown by some 10 per cent of Boder's sample, is one where sight vocabulary is small but word-attack skills are good. This 'dyseidetic' pattern suggests that visual skills are weak but phonological skills are intact. A further 30 per cent of Boder's sample showed severe dyslexic difficulties exemplified by a mixed dysphonetic–dyseidetic pattern. We have observed children with phonological disorder who display such a pattern. For example, an 11-year-old girl made the following reading errors after considering the target words for some seconds. She read 'command' as 'cabinet', 'purpose' as 'plimsoll' and 'hunger' as 'ham' which she then changed to 'gammon'. Clearly, these words were not in her sight vocabulary and she was unsuccessful with word-attack skills.

A second line of investigation involves the analysis of reading errors. It is important to include both regular (e.g. 'dance', 'fresh') and irregular (e.g. 'laugh', 'broad') words in a reading test because particular approaches to these words reveal different sorts of error. (See Appendix 1.) Both regular and irregular words can be read by a direct, visual approach but only regular words can be handled by a phonological strategy. The application of grapheme–phoneme rules to an irregular word will lead to a 'regularization' error, e.g. broad/brode, cough/koog–h, pint/pinnt (Coltheart, Masterson, Byng, Prior and Riddoch, 1983).

For these reasons a corpus of reading errors should be analysed for two sorts of error: regularization errors, as described above, and visual errors which share at least 50 per cent of letters with targets, irrespective of order (breath/bread, pint/print, organ/orange). An individual who makes a majority of regularization errors must be making use of a phonological strategy, while an individual who makes primarily visual errors may be relying upon visual or 'logographic' reading skills.

To illustrate this, Tim and Robin were two boys with specific learning difficulties. Both were of the same Reading Age, yet on simple tests of regular and irregular word reading, they performed differently. Tim read more regular than irregular words correctly (9 versus 5 out of 10). Robin read more irregular than regular words (5 versus 2 out of 10). These scores suggested that Tim could use phonological skills more proficiently than Robin. Indeed, this difference was borne out by the reading errors of the boys. Tim's errors were best characterized as regularizations: cough/cuff, move/muv, build/bald, aunt/a–unt, gone/known. Robin made no such errors. Most of his were visually similar to their targets: sign/sing, broad/boarder, sort/short, check/cheek.

So, an individual who shows a 'dyseidetic' approach to reading and who makes regularization errors has good phonological but weak visual skills. It should be noted that this type of individual has entered the alphabetic phase of literacy. An individual who shows a 'dysphonetic' approach and makes visual errors may be unable to apply phonological strategies. For dyslexic children who show this profile, reading will be arrested within the logographic phase and remedial intervention will be obligatory if progress is to be made.

Assessing phonological reading skill

To confirm the clinical impression than an individual has deficient phonological reading skill, it is possible to directly test knowledge of grapheme–phoneme correspondences. To begin with, a test in which an individual is asked to give the sounds of the letters of the alphabet, digraphs (ch, th, sh) and consonant blends (bl, dw, str) can be revealing. This should be followed by a test of nonword reading. Single syllable nonwords can be derived from real words by changing initial sounds (see Appendix 1). If a child has entered the alphabetic phase, the nonwords should be read almost as easily as equivalent real words. Tim (mentioned above) made only 2 out of 10 errors on a test of nonword reading. These were: darge/drag, sheck/shreck. In contrast, Robin was only able to read one nonword correctly. His errors were frequently real words bearing visual similarity to the nonwords: tresh/trash, hase/haze, darge/dragon, smade/swab, jang/jag.

It is important to sound a note of caution concerning the use of nonwords with dyslexic children who have already received intensive remediation. Tuition is frequently directed towards, and indeed results in, an improvement in phonic skill. In such cases a child may do well when asked to read simple nonwords. However, deficits may be revealed when two syllable versions are presented (Snowling, 1981). An example of a more complex nonword reading test is provided in Appendix 1.

The tests described so far can ascertain whether a child is functioning within the logographic or alphabetic phases for reading. To test at the orthograhic phase is really to test for an adult level of literacy. For this reason only a cursory discussion is called for. A quick test of orthographic knowledge involves reading and defining homophones (Coltheart *et al*, 1983). To explain briefly, an individual who does not confuse the meanings of visually similar words which sound the same (board/bored, fare/fair, son/sun, medal/meddle) must be able to make reference to detailed orthographic representations of printed words. Dyslexic individuals who have compensated for their reading difficulty seem to be able to make these distinctions but whether or not they have truly entered the orthographic phase remains a moot point. While they read homophones without difficulty, they frequently continue to confuse them when spelling.

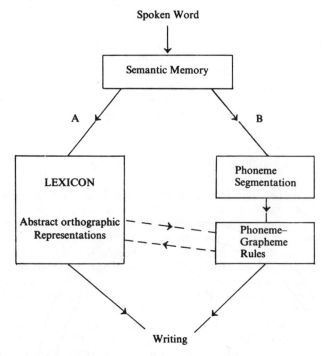

Figure 5.2 Information processing model of spelling process

Assessment of Spelling Strategies

The proficient adult speller can spell words automatically by directly addressing entries in the internal orthographic lexicon. This spelling process is depicted by route A, Figure 5.2. It has already been argued for reading that individuals within the orthographic phase retain strategies from earlier phases for use with unfamiliar words.

This is true of spelling also. Normal spellers can resort to a 'spelling by ear' strategy, depicted by route B, whenever it is useful to do so. Recent evidence suggests that this process is not truly 'alexical' as adult spellers sometimes spell nonwords by analogy with real words. For example, they spell 'yorl' as YALL, if preceded by BALL (Campbell, 1983). So it follows that there are links between the phoneme–grapheme rule system and the lexicon. This lexical influence is unlikely to be of significance prior to Reading Age 10 years when the child enters the orthographic phase (Campbell, in press). That is, not until reading experience furnishes the internal lexicon with detailed orthographic representations. Assessment of spelling strategies must examine not only orthographic knowledge (A). It must also investigate the functioning of the phonological spelling route (B) which can be used independently.

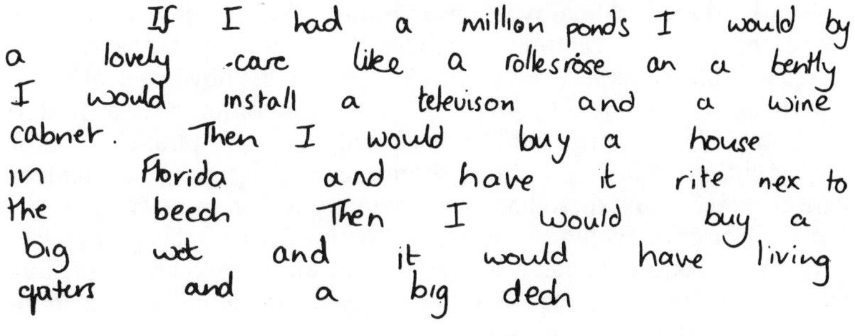

If I had a million ponds I would by
a lovely .care like a rollesröse an a bently
I would install a televison and a wine
cabnet. Then I would buy a house
in Florida and have it rite nex to
the beech Then I would buy a
big wot and it would have living
qaters and a big dech

Figure 5.3 Phonetic spelling from a teenage dyslexic

Assessment of spelling strategies has been traditionally carried out through error analysis. Important distinctions have been made between children who spell phonetically and those who make phonetically inaccurate errors (Boder, 1973; Nelson and Warrington, 1974; Sweeney and Rourke, 1978). A person whose spelling errors are primarily phonetic (see Figure 5.3) has good phonological spelling skill (Frith, 1980). There are no difficulties either with phoneme segmentation or with phoneme–grapheme rules, and therefore their deficit must be at lexical level. It could be argued that they have poor orthographic knowledge and therefore their spelling development is arrested within the alphabetic phase. A simple test of this hypothesis would involve the spelling of homophones. Individuals retaining alphabetic skills should confuse these words in spelling.

By contrast, individuals who make primarily nonphonetic spelling errors (see Figure 5.4) have difficulty in applying phonological spelling strategies. Their deficit may reside either with phoneme segmentation (B1) or with phoneme–grapheme translation (B2), and, as it often turns out, with both.

It is important when examining nonphonetic spelling errors to question whether they suggest segmentation problems or whether instead they reflect immaturities in the phonological processes. Analysis of the spelling of normal young children suggests that certain types of error are to be expected in terms of the child's development.

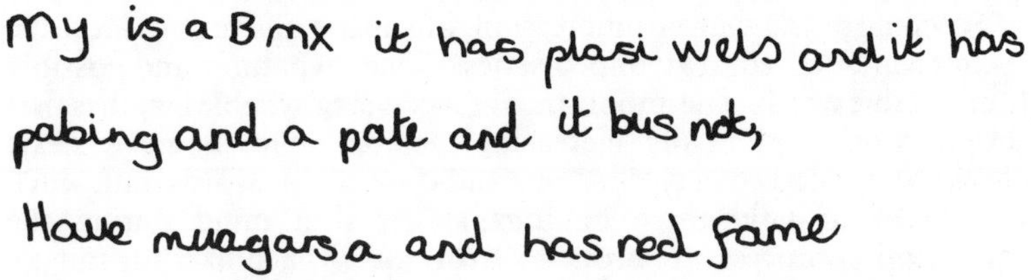

My is a Bmx it has plasi wels and it has
pabing and a pate and it bus not,
Have muagars a and has red fame

My (bike) is a BMX it has plastic wheels and it has padding and a plate and it does not have mudguards and has a red frame

Figure 5.4 Free writing from a 10-year-old who makes nonphonetic spelling errors

Firstly, there is difficulty in representing vowel sounds. Vowels are represented in a seemingly arbitrary way in English and it is unreasonable to expect a young child to have knowledge of these conventions. Up until Reading Age 9 years it is common for a child to 'mistranscribe' a vowel without necessarily having a phonological or segmentation 'deficit', e.g. bump/bomp, cigarette/cigerrit, contented/cantntid. Secondly, there has been some discussion in recent years of the tendency for spelling processes to reflect earlier speech processes (Marcel, 1980; Snowling, 1982). From this another common spelling error seen developmentally is the tendency to simplify consonant clusters in a rule-governed way, e.g.

instructed/instrucked

membership/mebership

contented/coteted.

Similarly, young spellers may often omit unstressed syllables, e.g.

cigarette/sigret

membership/membship.

Although, strictly speaking, these latter errors are nonphonetic, it would be incorrect to take them as signifying 'deficient' phonological skills because they occur during normal development. A child with a specific learning disability who displays a majority of these errors is likely to be developing normally, but slowly.

Therefore the assessment of spelling strategies is based upon error analysis. There are few hard and fast rules about how to elicit a corpus of errors. It is important to examine errors made in free writing as well as in dictation. Many children can spell reasonably well when all of their attention is devoted to the task. However, what will be important in their school experience will be to spell whilst also thinking, planning and developing ideas. In this situation, many more spelling errors are likely to occur and these must be examined during a comprehensive assessment.

To confirm the clinical impression which the above provides, the speller can be asked to attempt a series of one, two, three and possibly four syllable words. The importance of increasing syllable length is that this imposes a gradually increasing memory load. Some dyslexic children can succeed in spelling one and two syllable words, but, when they need to hold three or four syllables in mind during the transcription process, are prone to error. (See Appendix 1 for sample spelling test.) In short, spelling by ear involves phoneme segmentation, sound sequencing and auditory memory. Many dyslexic children find it difficult to apply phonological spelling strategies because of difficulties at one or other of these levels. Although they may enter the alphabetic phase for spelling, they find it difficult to perfect alphabetic skills. Indeed this may explain why they have difficulty transferring them to the reading situation.

It is interesting that there is often a connection between reading and spelling styles. Boder's dysphonetic dyslexics spelled in a nonphonetic manner whereas the dyseidetic group displayed an alphabetic approach. It will be recalled that earlier the contrasting reading styles of Tim and Robin were described. Robin had extreme difficulty with phonological reading strategies. His spelling errors reveal a corresponding difficulty with phonological spelling skills. When asked to spell one syllable words he did reasonably well, 6 out of 10 being phonetically correct. However, only 4 of his attempts at two syllable words were phonetically acceptable. The others reflected segmentation and/or sequencing problems:

polish/poleas

finger/thinger

trumpet/trupic

tulip/tyip

kitten/kintern.

When presented with three syllable words, Robin had no success whatsoever. The additional memory and sequencing load which these imposed compromised performance considerably:

contented/coled

membership/mander

September/saplder

adventure/anger

instructed/instruti.

Robin's reading and spelling development both appear to be arrested within the logographic phase. In contrast, Tim had entered the alphabetic phase for reading. His spelling reflected poor orthographic knowledge but no difficulty with phonological spelling strategies. One and two syllable words were all phonetically correct. Furthermore, his spellings of three syllable words all portrayed their syllabic structure correctly. Some were perfectly phonetic (catalogue/caterlog), while others contained normal phonological immaturities. These included simplifications of consonant clusters:

refreshment/refreschmet

instructed/intrukted

understand/undersand,

or difficulties with vowel transcription:

cigarette/cigerite

adventure/advinter.

It can therefore be concluded that Tim was functioning within the alphabetic phase but was still perfecting alphabetic skills. To some extent, he may have been awaiting further 'orthographic' experience before he could portray the sound structure of words perfectly.

Conclusions

It has been argued that reading and spelling are independent processes but that their development is interdependent. It follows that it is useful to consider written language difficulties within the context of reading and spelling development. As we have seen, different individuals encounter problems at different stages of the acquisition process. Children who (like Robin) have difficulties prior to the alphabetic phase have variously been described in the literature as auditory dyslexics (Johnson and Myklebust, 1967), dysphonetic dyslexics (Boder, 1973), reading and spelling retardates (Nelson and Warrington, 1974) and developmental phonological dyslexics (Seymour and McGregor, 1984). Children who, like Tim, have difficulties with orthographic knowledge have been described as visual dyslexics (Johnson and Myklebust, 1967), dyseidetic dyslexics (Boder, 1973), spelling-only retardates (Nelson and Warrington, 1974), developmental surface dyslexics (Coltheart *et al*, 1983) and morphemic dyslexics (Seymour and McGregor, 1984). It is reasonable to question whether this profusion of labels is warranted. Standardized tests are important for determining whether or not a child has a specific learning disability. Nonstandard procedures are useful for determining possible reasons for the 'unexpected' failure of children with specific difficulties, but, more importantly, they allow us to identify their individual teaching needs.

Appendix 1

Lists of irregular, regular and nonwords for reading aloud.

Irregular	Regular	Nonwords	Complex Nonwords
laugh	fresh	tresh	tegwop
break	treat	freat	pedbim
sign	base	hase	jenter
broad	dance	hance	rasgan
cough	barge	darge	malzen
glove	spade	smade	romsig
move	kept	rept	molsmit
build	check	sheck	baltrid
aunt	sort	nort	venstor
gone	gang	jang	holtcom
			duncren
			kepstud

Lists of one, two and three syllable words for spelling.

One syllable	Two syllable	Three syllable
pet	apple	membership
lip	puppy	cigarette
cap	packet	catalogue
fish	trumpet	September
sack	kitten	adventure
tent	traffic	contented
trap	collar	refreshment
bump	tulip	instructed
nest	polish	umbrella
bank	finger	understand

Joy Stackhouse

6 Segmentation, Speech and Spelling Difficulties

Theoretical developments over the last few years have placed reading and spelling problems firmly within the field of language disorder (Vellutino, 1979). The relationship between specific reading difficulties and early language problems has been well documented (Ingram, Mason and Blackburn, 1970; Rutter and Yule, 1973) and increasingly speech therapists are becoming involved in the management of written language difficulties. It would be misleading however to imply that all speech disordered children will have similar problems – those that do may be vulnerable for different reasons.

Of particular interest is the comparison of children whose speech difficulty is phonetic in nature with those whose speech problem is associated with a difficulty within the phonological system. In the case of a phonetic difficulty, speech is distorted, often because of some structural abnormality (such as cleft palate) or a neurological impairment (such as dysarthria) but the system by which sounds are mapped onto meanings (internally) is essentially normal. In contrast, children with phonological difficulties do not always mark different meanings with the appropriate phonemic contrasts (e.g. they may say 'tea' for tea, key and see). In the serious cases, such as verbal dyspraxia, a mixed phonetic and phonological disorder exists and there may be no systematic relationship between speech sounds and meaning. A word pronounced correctly on one occasion may be misarticulated another time or a word may have many mispronunciations in an attempt to reach the target. In the face of such inconsistency, reading and spelling difficulties are to be anticipated since written language will be laid down onto a faulty spoken language base.

As an initial attempt to investigate the nature of reading and spelling processes in children with phonetic and phonological speech problems, two groups of children were tested (Stackhouse, 1982). The first group comprised cleft palate children ranging in age from 6 years 8 months to 11 years 4 months, while the second were a verbal dyspraxic group ranging in age from 7 years 3 months to 11 years 3 months. A group of normally speaking children were also tested.

The cleft palate children whose speech difficulties were primarily phonetic in nature were not significantly different to age matched normal children on reading and spelling tests. However, the dyspraxic group experienced greater difficulty. It became apparent that they were unable to utilize a sound by sound approach to reading unfamiliar words. The reading errors of cleft palate children suggested the use of a sound building strategy, e.g. 'sabre' was read as ['seɪbri] and 'ceiling' was read as ['kɛ[ɪŋ]. In contrast, the dyspraxic children's errors could be described as illogical, e.g. 'canary' was read as 'competition', 'dream' as 'under'. These responses seemed to be guesses cued by individual letters within the words. To confirm that the dyspraxic children were unable to decode using letter–sound rules, they were administered a silent test of phonology (Coltheart, 1980). The children were asked to sort cards into same and different piles. Each card showed two words which either sounded the same when read (silently) or sounded different, e.g. fid/phid or fid/prid. As one might expect, the performance of normal children on this task correlated with reading age. This was also true for the cleft palate group. However, amongst dyspraxic children, reading age increased without a corresponding increase in performance on the silent test of phonology. It could be argued that the dyspraxic group were increasing their reading age by reliance on a visual reading strategy in the absence of phonological skill. To this extent, they were performing in the same way as the dyslexic children discussed by Snowling (1980).

The spelling of the dyspraxic children was also qualitatively different from that seen in cleft palate and normal groups. The latter children made primarily phonetic spelling errors – they spelled words as they sounded, e.g. sooner/soona, might/mit, boat/bot. In contrast, errors made by the dyspraxic children were bizarre and they did not follow the normal processes identified in spelling development (Read, 1971; Chomsky, 1971), e.g. year/andere, health/heens, slippery/greid. In a separate study, children described as 'phonologically disordered' were also reported to make bizarre spelling errors (Robinson, Beresford and Dodd, 1982).

These studies suggest that children with an underlying phonological disability are more at risk as far as reading and spelling difficulties are concerned than those with a phonetic speech difficulty. It is recognized, however, that children in the latter group may be vulnerable and could well show delayed development of written language skills because of poor health, hospitalization and through missing school. Nonetheless, the incidence of difficulties *specific* to written language should be lower in children with phonetic speech problems than in those who have phonological disorders.

So far, discussion has been concerned with reading and spelling performance. However, profiles collected from speech disordered populations make clear that these children are most at risk of having spelling difficulties. It would be incorrect to consider reading and spelling as the same process moving in opposite directions. A clear dissociation between the two has been demonstrated in both young children (Bradley and Bryant, 1979) and adolescents (Frith, 1980). Bradley and Bryant found that both normal and backward readers could read words which they could not spell and spell words which they could not read. In an adolescent group Frith demonstrated that, in spite of reading well, unexpected spelling problems occurred. This pattern is frequently seen at a younger age in speech disordered groups. R.A., for example, had a mild phonological difficulty and although his reading age was in line with chronological age (9 years) his spelling age was only 7 years 7 months.

Why Might Children with Speech Disorders have Reading and Spelling Difficulties?

The dissociations within written language development make sense in the light of current theories. In order to appreciate the reasons for the speech disordered groups' vulnerability to reading and spelling difficulties it is useful to consider two current models of reading and spelling.

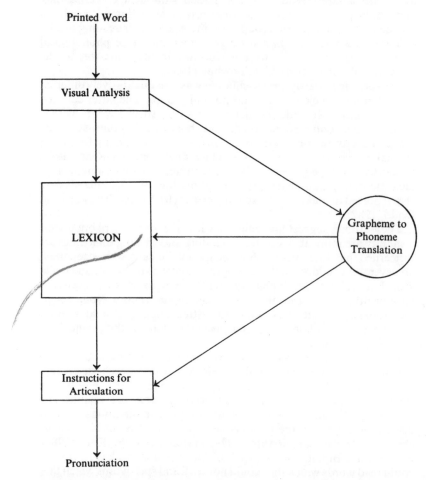

Figure 6.1 Two-route model of the reading process (after Coltheart, 1980)

First, Coltheart's (1980) model of single word reading shows that there are two routes to meaning – the direct route (visual) which would be used to read a familiar word such as 'cat' or a learned irregular word such as 'yacht', and the indirect route (phonological) used for unfamiliar regular words such as 'utopianism' and nonsense words such as 'lembot'. (See Figure 6.1.)

In the normal development of reading, children first acquire a sight vocabulary through the direct route and then learn phoneme–grapheme correspondences, so acquiring the phonological strategy of reading via the indirect route. This strategy is necessary for reading development – without it new words cannot be tackled and reading can only progress up to the limits of visual memory (see Snowling, this volume).

To a certain extent, using predominantly the direct route can be successful since reading is primarily a recognition process. This explains why the dyspraxic group referred to earlier could increase their reading age without developing the phonological route to reading – as demonstrated by their poor performance on the silent test of phonology in which nonwords had to be sorted as to whether they sounded the same (aif/afe) or different (aif/ait). Unfortunately, as spelling is a retrieval process (Frith, 1980), the visual route can no longer sustain them. They are forced to use a phonological route (see Figure 6.2) and hence have marked difficulty. Snowling and Stackhouse (1983) argued that the spelling problems of the dyspraxic children they studied could not be explained by poor knowledge of letter forms, visual copying problems or poor articulation. No one to one relationship existed between speech and spelling errors. However, great difficulty in segmenting the word prior to spelling was noted. For example, 'Pam' was repeated correctly, segmented as 'pe–te' and spelled 'potm'. 'Nick' was also repeated correctly, segmented as 'ke–ke–ne–i–te' and spelled 'cat'.

Applying these data to the second theoretical model, Frith's (1980) model of (indirect) spelling (see Figure 6.2), it can be seen that such errors arise early on in the spelling process, namely at the stage where speech sounds are analysed prior to phoneme–grapheme translation. Children whose spelling errors are phonetic, e.g. 'catalog' for 'catalogue', break down further on in this process even though they cannot yet select the conventionally correct graphemes to portray the phonemes they have segmented.

In summary, children with persisting speech disorders of a phonological nature often learn to use the direct route in reading but not the indirect route. Since their knowledge of grapheme–phoneme correspondences is reduced, they are particularly at risk of spelling difficulties as spelling explicitly requires such knowledge. These children often present with a profile of poor auditory processing skills and breakdown on sound segmentation tasks. These difficulties further exacerbate their spelling problems. Thus, they frequently show a specific phonological dyslexia accompanied by phonological dysgraphia. This syndrome, sometimes called dysphonetic dyslexia (Boder, 1973), is far more common among children with a history of speech difficulties than is a reading difficulty associated with visual perceptual problems. However, it should be recognized that children may have a mixed disability, both visual and phonological, and that individual differences are inevitably found. From such rationale and clinical experience, the following assessment and management procedures have been developed.[1]

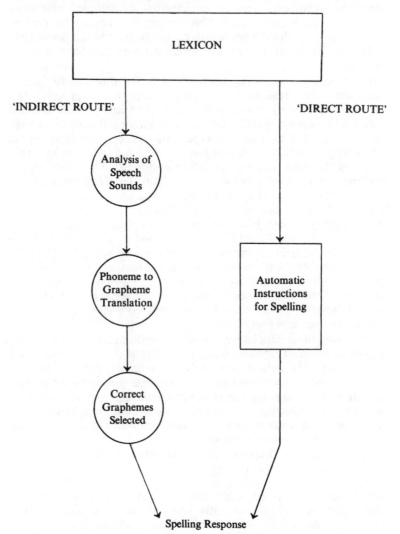

Figure 6.2 Model of the spelling process (after Frith, 1980)

[1] In conjunction with Maggie Snowling and John Rack at University College London.

What Should We Assess?

It is assumed that all children referred to a speech therapist will have a full verbal language assessment in addition to the assessments outlined here. (See Klein, this volume.) Fluency also needs to be carefully monitored. Many young 'stammerers' present with language problems and later show reading and spelling difficulties.

The aims of the assessment procedures to be described are not only to analyse the symptoms of the problem, i.e. the speech, reading and spelling errors, but also to investigate the underlying nature of the problem and to identify the strengths and weaknesses in the child's cognitive processing.

Speech

It is beyond the scope of this paper to discuss methods of speech assessment in detail but an outline will be given. It is now recognized that a simple Initial/Medial/Final sound substitution assessment is not helpful when working with persisting speech disorders (Carney, 1979; Grunwell, 1980) and that fuller phonetic and phonological procedures are necessary (Weiner, 1979; Ingram, 1981; Crystal, 1982; Grunwell – in press).

A useful speech assessment should include:

a) A standardized articulation test to establish an age level for comparison with other skills tested; for example, the Edinburgh Articulation Test (Anthony, Bogle, Ingram and McIsaac, 1971).

b) An oral examination of structure and movement.

c) Isolated articulatory tasks such as repetition of sounds and diadochokinetic rates (Canning and Rose, 1974; Fletcher, 1978).

d) Combination of sounds in syllables and words involving phonetic place change, e.g. pop, tap, peck. (For further guidelines on use of phonetic context in discrimination and production tasks, the reader is referred to Fleming, 1971.)

e) Imitation versus spontaneous speech tasks.

f) Rating of intelligibility in spontaneous speech.

g) Phonological output assessment of sounds in syllable initial and final position in one and two syllable words, e.g. /d/ in day, daddy, head, bedtime.

h) Description of speech errors in three to five syllable real and nonsense words, e.g. spaghetti/skapedi, caterpillar/pakerlitter, hippopotamus/pitohomapus.

i) Recognition and production of prosodic changes in words, e.g. [' ɛbədi] vs. [ə' bɛdi] vs. [əbə' di], and in phrases, e.g. *Look!* over there vs. Look over *there*. More general moods can also be manipulated, e.g. angry, happy.

j) Phonological knowledge and awareness is currently receiving much attention but is often overshadowed by phonological output tasks in assessment procedures. Coltheart's (1980) silent test of phonology discussed previously is useful in that it isolates phonological coding from articulatory performance as no verbal response is required. Moving on to morphophonological knowledge, Hughes' (1983) procedure (following Berko, 1958) of requesting the plural ending of real (e.g. mouse) vs. nonsense words (e.g. wug) can examine the internalization of morphophonological rules. The child's awareness of his own errors also should be investigated. Hughes' procedure again might be followed. She suggests that by using familiar pictures the tester can ask the child 'Is this a ....?', either producing the word correctly or imitating the child's form. Howell and Dean (1983) have discussed the role of phonological awareness in therapy but the field of meta linguistics is not limited to the speech assessment. It incorporates auditory processing and a more general awareness of cognitive processes and strategies, for example, knowing the most efficient method of problem solving. (For a further discussion of meta skills the reader is referred to Van Kleek [1981].)

Auditory skills

AUDITORY DISCRIMINATION

Speech disordered children will often pass auditory discrimination tests such as in the Aston Index (Newton and Thomson, 1976) or the Wepman (1958), where a same/different judgement has to be made on verbally presented pairs of words, e.g. gate–gate, big–big. By using the same procedure but with more complex nonwords, e.g. bikut–bituk, besket–bekset, preliminary findings suggest that children with persisting speech problems around the age of 11 years might be below the level expected for their chronological age.

Errors have been noted on place change (g/d), high frequency sounds (f/s), cluster sequences (sk/ks), and sound transpositions (ibikus–ikibus). There is therefore some indication that our routine tests of auditory discrimination may not be sophisticated enough to detect problems of input phonology in the older child and require further attention.

Therapists might develop their own tests of auditory discrimination by manipulating syllable number and cluster complexity. Paired nonsense words can be devised which transpose sounds in clusters, e.g. wesp/weps or syllables, e.g. retuk/rekut.

Poor auditory memory is a well known feature in speech disordered and dyslexic children. Digit span tests such as included in the Illinois Test of Psycholinguistic Abilities – I.T.P.A. (Kirk, McCarthy and Kirk, 1968) and the Aston Index will confirm this. K.F., aged 14 years, for example, has persisting articulatory and spelling difficulties. His auditory memory is contained to five digits forwards and three digits backwards. Any child with poor auditory memory will find phonological coding difficult and be at risk of spelling problems. In such cases further investigation of auditory organization and segmentation skills are required.

AUDITORY ORGANIZATION

Bradley and Bryant (1983) have highlighted the importance of the ability to organize and categorize speech sounds when learning to read and spell. Children's performance in the pre-school years on odd one out tasks as in: 'sun gun rub fun' or 'lot cot pot hat', or 'bud bun bus rug', was found to be predictive of their reading and spelling performance at 8 years of age.

The report on findings with speech disordered children will come as no surprise. Using the Bradley Test of Auditory Organisation (1980) with secondary school age children, performance was often at the 5 year level or below. L.B., for example, a 15-year-old boy with severe phonological difficulties in speech, reading and spelling, performed at less than five year level on this test.

Rhyme detection and production

As many of the speech disordered children seen have had reduced auditory memory and are unable to remember the items in the Bradley test, a more simple rhyme detection task which can be presented both visually and auditorially has been devised. This involves the presentation of a target word or picture, e.g. 'purse', followed by two others, one of which will rhyme with the target, e.g. 'nurse', while the other is either a semantically related distractor, e.g. 'bag', or an alliteration of the target, e.g. 'peas'. The child is asked to select from the pair the one that rhymes with the target. Normal 6-year-olds and some 5-year-olds were found to be at ceiling on this task. It is therefore possible to detect a delay in rhyming skills in the clinical population. Older speech disordered children have made errors on this task equivalent to much younger children. For example, C.G., aged 8 years 5 months, who has a mild speech and learning difficulty and M.C., aged 10 years 7 months, who has a severe speech and learning difficulty, both scored below the five year level on this test. It should be noted from these examples that the severity of the speech problem is not necessarily indicative of the severity of the segmentation difficulties.

Rhyme production tasks will also expose difficulties (Stackhouse and Snowling, 1983). Although performance can be erratic in the preschool years, children as young as 3 or 4 years can produce rhymes spontaneously in their play, even though they are not necessarily aware of the concept of rhyme. To illustrate the possible severity of the problem, responses in a rhyme production task from L.B. will be compared with a control child.

S.M. is a normal speaking 5-year-old in a reception class and L.B. is a 15-year-old developmental dyspraxic in a language unit attached to a normal school.

Target	Response	
	S.M.	**L.B.**
pig	mig, kig	peg, pack
key	pea, tea, me	king
hat	mat, cat, bat	hen

L.B. had no concept of rhyme but had received phonics teaching which may explain the above alliterations to the target. He has a severe auditory organization difficulty as seen in his poor performance on the Bradley and rhyming tests, but has shown some indication of sound knowledge by his alliterative errors.

The persistence of semantic associations is indicative of a more severe problem in auditory organization. Such associations are common in the normal nursery school child but should not persist through to the school years. C.F., aged 11 years 9 months, has a severe speech difficulty and poor organization skills. She produced the following associations in a rhyme production task:

Target	Response
comb	brush
shell	sea
sun	tan
wool	cotton

It is recommended that more than one response is requested from the child. Often the speech disordered child is unable to retain the rhyming strategy even if initially successful. M.C., for example, aged 10 years 7 months, shows this 'free floating' use of rhyme, alliteration and semantic associations in the following:

Target	*Response*
map	train, map, trap, hatch, mat, mop
sur	lun, mun, clouds, sky
bed	bacon, bread, blackboard

Syllable and phoneme segmentation

Beating syllables and rhythms on musical instruments and table tops has been a popular therapy activity for many years. It makes acoustic sense that syllable segmentation precedes sound segmentation as the latter is contaminated by the dynamic nature of coarticulations. The more salient syllable divisions are marked by peaks of acoustic energy.

For guidelines in assessment, studies have found that 90 per cent of normal 6-year-old children were accurate when tapping out the number of syllables in a word, and only 70 per cent were accurate when tapping out phonemes (Liberman, Shankweiler, Fischer and Carter, 1974). Therapists and teachers will know that problems persist beyond this age in children with speech and written language difficulties.

N.P., aged 7 years 6 months, was referred to speech therapy because of his 'stammer'. He was at chance level only when beating syllables and had no concept of phoneme segmentation in games like 'I-Spy'. When asked to find something in the room beginning with 'd', he looked round intently and responded 'd–floor, d–window, d–telephone'. Furthermore investigation showed him to be a poor reader, who could only 'spell' his first name.

Phoneme segmentation tasks are varied. Focus may be on counting the number of sounds or identifying/producing sounds in specific word positions. Sound blending as well as analysis should be included (the Aston Index and I.T.P.A. are again referred to).

Segmentation tasks will need to be graded in terms of difficulty. Perin's (1983) spoonerism task in which the initial phonemes of two names must be switched, e.g. 'Bad Manners' – Mad Banners', has proved quite impossible for speech disordered children. Those who have attempted it have taken longer than expected from normal data to transpose the initial sounds and have often made errors. K.F., aged 14 years 11 months, for example, was slow in his responses and often vocalized the sounds he was transposing, e.g. Chuck Berry – [ʧ ʧ bʌk ʤ deɪ' ʤeɪvi], or simply gave up, e.g. Jethro Tull – Joe Tull. This only happened towards the end of the test and shows how quickly these children fatigue compared to non-speech-handicapped groups who do not need to make such an effort in order to accomplish the task. A simplified version of spoonerisms using CVC syllables, e.g. 'fat dog', might be attempted.

Reading

Reading comprehension and expression need to be assessed. The Neale Analysis of Reading Ability can be used to examine prose reading and comprehension. Routine administration of the Aston Index to all speech disordered children over five years of age will ensure a check on phoneme–grapheme naming and single word reading through the Schonell Test. (See Augur, this volume.) As children may not get very far with this test, the Carver Word Recognition Test is recommended for beginner readers or older children with severe problems. It also provides more qualitative information on the errors produced. Caution is needed when interpreting results from tests such as the Schonell Graded Word Reading Test, given that children may show age appropriate performance by relying on the visual route even when a deficit exists in the phonological route to reading (Snowling, 1980; Stackhouse, 1982).

Returning to Coltheart's (1980) model of single word reading, Snowling (this volume) suggests ways of evaluating the efficiency of both the visual and phonological routes. In order to illustrate this procedure, the assessment profile of one speech disordered child will be discussed. C.F. is 12 years and 7 months old with a Reading Age of 7 years and 9 months. She has a severe speech difficulty of a phonetic and phonological nature and attends a language unit attached to a normal school.

A qualitative analysis of her single word reading revealed a reliance on the visual route. Visual errors, as a result of overloading her visual memory system, made up 20 per cent of her errors, e.g. plug → plum, ward → word. No regularization errors were found, i.e. irregular words were never pronounced letter by letter, e.g. wand → [wænd].

A high proportion of errors in the speech disordered group have been found to be unsuccessful sound attempts. Often the children have been taught to use a sounding out strategy in school but because of a specific deficit in sound analysis and synthesis, they are unable to reach the target. Approximately 40 per cent of C.F.'s errors showed this pattern and usually resulted in a 'don't know' response. For example,

bleat → [bə bə ḷe'ɪt
  'ɪtɪn'ɪtɪn
  bə'leɪ
  'bleɪ'ɪtɪn]

Another test for use of the phonological route is to compare reading performance of regular and irregular words. Normal children can read regular words more easily than irregular as they can utilize a sounding out strategy to attack unfamiliar regular words. For example, D.A, whose Reading Age is 7 years 7 months, could read 55 per cent of regular words presented but only 23 per cent of irregular words. C.F. also read 23 per cent of the irregular words but showed no significant improvement when reading regular words.

The most obvious way of testing the use of the phonological route is to present the child with unfamiliar regular words or nonsense words. C.F. was unable to read any such words. Errors appeared to be unsuccessful sound attempts, e.g. spake → [skæt], garket → ['golɪk], tatch → [tə'læk].

There is therefore a clear indication that children like C.F. have difficulties with phonological reading strategies. This is accompanied by poor auditory organization and segmentation skills. In the case of C.F., for example, her performance on such tasks was around the five year level.

Spelling

In order to quantify the extent of the problem and compare performance with other abilities, a standardized assessment will again be a starting point. The Schonell Graded Spelling Test (included in the Aston Index) will provide a spelling age and data for qualitative analysis. Clumsy children or those with poor handwriting skills will benefit from using plastic letters or letter cards.

When analysing spelling errors the speech therapist should utilize the skills she has developed in her phonological analysis of children's speech since a similar procedure can be followed.

Firstly, normal simplifying processes in the spelling system should be identified. If present in an older child they may be indicative of delayed development. For example, many beginning spellers confuse the short vowels, 'i, e, a'; reduce clusters – particularly nasals, e.g. bank → bak, and delete unstressed syllables. Many will confuse letter sound and name, e.g. boat → bot, or stress the letter sound with exaggerated aspiration which is realized as an intrusive 'e' or 'u', e.g. boat → beot or bote. The first step when analysing spelling errors is therefore to isolate what might be considered normal even if delayed, just as in a speech assessment.

Secondly, errors directly associated with the speech pattern can be identified. For example, J.M., aged 8 years 5 months, had persisting voice/voiceless confusion in both speech and spelling, e.g. pin → bin, two → do, cap → gap. K.F., aged 11 years, had particular difficulty with the 'wrly' group of sounds in speech and spelt 'library' as 'libily' and 'slippery' as 'sliply'. R.A., aged 9 years, still uses /f/ for /θ/ and /v/ for /ð/. Interestingly this pattern was reversed in his spelling, e.g. traffic → trathic, finger → thinger, nerve → nerth. These three examples of children with intelligible speech but residual difficulties constitute the most common sound errors reflected in spelling. It is stressed, however, that in the more complex and persisting speech problems no such clear relationship between the speech and spelling errors has been found.

R.A.'s performance on spelling words of increasing length (Snowling, this volume) shows the importance of including more difficult tasks in the assessment procedure in order to provoke a diagnosis. The use of multisyllabic words will force children to rely on a phonetic strategy for words that they do not know. According to Frith's (1980) model, if they are successful at stage one – segmentation – the resulting spelling will sound correct when read back, e.g. collar → koler, but will not obey the rules of English spelling. If sound segmentation prior to phoneme–grapheme translation is a problem, the errors will appear bizarre, e.g. instructed → nisokder.

On initial assessment, R.A. appeared to be delayed in his spelling development. He was 80 per cent accurate on the spelling of single syllable words and showed immature errors, e.g. bump → bomp. He also coped up to a point with increased syllable load and attempted phoneme–grapheme matching, e.g. cigarette → sigaret, but when cluster complexity was added to syllable length, he showed errors of a more serious phonological nature, e.g. discovery → dicoary, and even lost the syllable count, e.g. umbrella → upbla. As would now be predicted, he was found to be poor on auditory organization tasks even though he has age appropriate reading.

Fortunately for R.A., only a small number of his errors were phonologically disordered. Other children seen, however, have had a predominance of these, e.g. refreshment → lpohet. Such errors are typical of children with persisting speech problems. At first they may appear 'bizarre' or random but drawing the parallel with speech assessment, time spent analysing the atypical patterns often reveals a system, even if somewhat idiosyncratic. M.C., for example, is unable to segment the sounds particularly when clusters are involved. He does however persevere with this strategy and records most of his attempts:

um/bre/lla – r/berh/er/rel/r a/r l/srlll/es
1   2   3   2   2   2   3   2 2   2   3

Note that focus is on the stressed syllable and that breakdown is at the cluster even though in this case the r/l sound order is retained.

C.F., whose reading profile was discussed earlier, shows a different approach when she tries to spell by previously learned word compo- nents, e.g. refreshment → withfirstmint; adventure → andbackself. She seems to have abandoned the sound segmentation approach and certainly did have difficulties with this.

It is therefore important to go further than a standardized test of spelling. Quality of errors needs to be investigated and the child's total behaviour when spelling should be monitored. Speed of response (even when correct) as well as strategies used, e.g. subvocal segmentation, should be recorded. Written language and spelling errors in continuous writing will also need to be examined.

Awareness of reading and spelling strategies

Using the questionnaire suggested by Francis (1982), children were asked to reflect on their reading and spelling strategies. M.C., you will recall, has a serious segmentation difficulty but believed that 'sounding out' a word *always* helped him to read it. Given that the majority of his errors were unsuccessful sound attempts, it becomes apparent that he had little awareness of the reading process.

Other children have shown insight into their difficulties and have tried to develop compensatory techniques. K.F., for example, at 14 years 11 months of age stated that in order to spell unfamiliar words he would 'listen for the sharpest notes then try to think of a word like it.' He also has difficulty with sound segmentation but appears to be tuning into a large unit – the syllable. This may go some way in explaining C.F.'s spelling by word components, cited above, and highlights the importance of listening to the children's reports on their reading and spelling behaviour.

In summary, having identified through the assessment:

(a) a profile of ability on speech, language, reading and spelling tests
(b) the level and modality of breakdown
(c) the severity of the difficulties and their manifestations in 'real life'
(d) the coping strategies adopted

then remediation can be planned.

How Can Speech Therapists Help?

Although many of the skills worked on in speech therapy sessions for the purpose of increasing intelligibility are the same as those required for the development of reading and spelling, the small jump needed in order to work on speech and spelling in synchrony is often not made. It is a pity if the work carried out in the clinical setting and the classroom are isolated when there is such a high degree of compatibility.

For the purpose of this chapter the management focus will be on speech and auditory processing, although it is recognized that some children may also require work on visual perception and organization. Handwriting should be included in a management programme and language skills cannot be separated from the following suggestions (see Klein, this volume).

Firstly, possible tools and techniques will be examined and then, secondly, suggestions will be made as to activities and games, with the aim of linking speech with reading and spelling activities. Finally, timing of intervention will be discussed.

Tools and techniques

PHONEME–GRAPHEME MATCHED CARDS

Many of the speech disordered children seen have a mixed phonetic and phonological disability and require training in articulating and contrasting sounds (Stackhouse, 1984). For this purpose sound cards where pictures represent sounds have proved very popular. Tradition, however, has given us rather unfortunate phoneme–grapheme confused pictures to represent speech sounds, e.g. fish for /p/, gun for /k/; perhaps we should look no further than this as to why children in speech therapy clinics persist in their use of the stopping process and confuse voice/voiceless sounds!

In the light of criticism from teachers over the clash with reading schemes, such as the pictogram system, the redrawing of picture cards would seem a minor change to make in what is a useful and versatile therapy tool.

Therapists may like to consider the following system where the sound made corresponds with the grapheme:

p – pipe	f – fan
b – ball	v – van
t – tap	s – snake
d – drum	z – zip
k – kick	
g – gun	

The velar sounds have always been particularly difficult. In the above system /k/ can be described as a kicking sound and /g/ for gun lends itself to sounding more like a machine gun than /k/ ever did. /ʃ/ can still be denoted by a gesture or picture of 'be quiet' as it stands as a unit of meaning in its own right. The remaining sounds /ʤ, r, l, w, j, θ/ can be represented by oral diagrams or the grapheme, as it is unlikely that these sounds would be involved in the pre-school programme anyway.

Through this concordance therapists allow themselves the opportunity of working *simultaneously* on speech and segmentation skills.

COLOUR CODED SYSTEMS

Another popular tool in therapy sessions is the use of colour codes as a visual reminder of language structures (Lea, 1970) or of sound groups (Kellet *et al*, 1984).

As there are a variety of such codes being used, both published and spontaneous, it is important not to mix them or clash with a system being taught in the school. For example, a therapist may have difficulties fitting her own colour coded speech programme into an equivalent coded syntax scheme. She may then turn to an alternative gestural cueing for the sounds, e.g. drawing thumb and index finger together for bilabials, or flicking index finger across thumb as in 'kicking' for velar plosive sounds.

Whatever method is used, the aim is to increase articulatory awareness when speaking and reading. Montgomery (1981) has reported that dyslexic children have poor awareness of articulation processes compared to normal children. Colour coding when coupled with articulatory and handwriting skills can contribute to the multisensory approach to teaching (see Augur, this volume).

It has been found useful to adopt a colour code in conjunction with a diacritic scheme in order to contrast voice, place and manner in speech reading and spelling. Adopting a traffic light analogy, all stop sounds are RED while continuants are GREEN. By playing with red and green groups, sound categorization games are introduced which can be linked with the stopping process in phonological work. To tackle place, diacritics are used. Underneath each grapheme an articulatory cue can be drawn; for example, teeth under 'f', lips under 'p', alveolar ridge under 't', velum under 'k'. Younger children may prefer to continue to use the symbol discussed earlier, e.g. a pipe under 'p' instead of lips, and this is further argument for matching phonemes and graphemes. By denoting place in some way, the phonological process of fronting can be worked on as well as alphabetic representation and articulatory skills.

Finally, voicing is often a persisting problem. 'Loud', i.e. voicing, can be marked by the cartoon symbol for 'bang', e.g. b . This system results in portraying phonetic differences between sounds, for example /p/ and /b/ are both red, with lips underneath them but /b/ has the additional voicing symbol over it. /t/ /s/ differ only in colour, while /d/ /g/ differ only in the place diacritic.

Sounds are therefore represented visually in letter form but with additional cues for voicing, place of articulation and manner of production. This allows for phonetic and phonological organization and can lead to segmentation activities with children compiling their own puzzle books of such games.

This system has also been adapted for work with adult patients and it is outlined here as a possible tool to be used in part or whole for appropriate patients.

Another system which may be used with speech disordered children is the Edith Norrie Letter Case. It was devised earlier this century by Edith Norrie (herself a dyslexic) to teach spelling and incorporates an articulatory awareness element. This time, colour is used to denote vowels from consonants and voicing. As each vowel is red, children learn not to select too many letters for a word without a red splash. It therefore helps with syllable segmentation. Voiced letters are green and voiceless black. Place of articulation is dealt with by the box presentation of the letters. The section on the left is labial, the middle is palatal and alveolar, and the right is velar. Punctuation cards are included as is a small mirror for feedback on oral movements. Although colour must not be confused, diacritics or symbols to denote place can be used in conjunction with this letter case and similar sound categorization games can be developed.

Now that some tools of work have been defined, suggestions will be given for some activities and the rationale behind them examined.

Activities

SOUND CATEGORIZATION

Bradley and Bryant (1983) have shown that there is a strong relationship between sound categorization training and learning to read and spell. In their study, 65 children who were non-readers and below average on sound categorization when starting school were chosen for an investigation of efficacy of training methods. The group was divided into four, those who
   1) received sound categorization tasks, e.g. listening for shared letters in paired words (hen/hat, hen/man).
   2) also received the above, but in addition were shown how each sound was represented in the alphabet by using plastic letters.
Groups (3) and (4) were controls.
   3) was taught semantic categorization, e.g. hen/pig are farm animals, hen/bat are animals.
   4) received no training.
Training took place in 40 individual sessions over two years. At the end of this time groups (1) and (2) were ahead of group (3). The greatest success in terms of reading and spelling skills was in group (2) which suggests a need for explicit teaching on alphabetic knowledge in addition to sound categorization. It is therefore suggested that, when using sound cards as discussed in the previous section, the grapheme is also present on the card and a multisensory approach is utilized. For more information on the tasks used, the reader is referred to Bradley (1980).

SYLLABLE AND PHONEME SEGMENTATION

Problems here may be early warning signs of the 'at risk' child. The speech therapist is likely to be one of the first contacts with the child through referral because of unintelligible speech or language and/or fluency difficulties and will therefore be influential in preparing the child for school. Work can begin early on syllable segmentation, e.g. copying beats; 'reading' beats from patterns; guessing how many beats in a word, and providing a word for a given number of beats. Alongside this, prosodic work can be introduced, e.g. stress patterns where the child can experiment with changing the emphasized beat in words and sentences. Children with dyspraxic speech problems have been found in need of extra help with this. (Edwards, 1982.)

   Phoneme segmentation is an inevitable component of articulation and phonological therapy. Isolating the first sound is usually easier than the final or vowel sounds. Phoneme segmentation games can be programmed from easy to hard and need not necessarily require a verbal response. Techniques normally employed are closed questions, forced alternatives and, finally, open questions (e.g. Does 'cat' begin with [k] – Yes/No? Does 'cat' begin with /k/ or /t/? What does 'cat' begin with?). Similarly, comparisons can be made on a Yes/No level, e.g. Does 'cat' begin with the same sound as 'can' (or 'hat')? Eventually the child can be asked to think of or find words/pictures beginning or ending with the same sound as the target.

There is only space to give general ideas on phoneme segmentation activities. For a further critical view of the use and range of phonemic awareness training tasks the reader is referred to Lewkowicz (1980).

RHYMING

Because of the strong correlation between the ability to rhyme, read and spell, rhyming experience should be a main focus of therapy in the pre-school years onwards. The speech therapist has an important prophylactic role in nursery schools and early language groups. Early activities can include 'Guess what I'm thinking' games giving clues such as 'It rhymes with dish and it swims' or 'It rhymes with moon and you use it to eat your pudding'. 'I went shopping and bought –' or 'I went on my holidays and took –' can generate rhyme strings, and rhyme tables and charts are to be encouraged. Attention needs also to be given to rhyme detection, e.g. finding rhyming pictures or rhyming words hidden in complex pictures, as well as rhyme production, e.g. what rhymes with – ?

Later these rhyming activities can be developed into chunking words into 'families', e.g. – eat, or – at words, which links with phoneme segmentation. 'Animal bodies' is often a good concrete start for such activities, where the head, body and tail correspond to the structure of CVC words. By decapitating a cat, for example, children can play with a variety of initial phonemes taken from other heads of animals so that a pig's head on a cat's body will say 'pat' while a horse's head will say 'hat'!

Graphemes can be used to replace heads and many rhyming words, both real and nonsense, can be generated. Nonwords have been found to be a strange concept to some speech disordered children and it may be necessary to work on this difference. Needless to say, equally gory games can be devised with tails and bodies and these will be left to the therapist's imagination!

It is hoped that the link between such sound categorization tasks and phonological therapy is becoming very clear. The principle of searching for patterns of processes and rules applies to both. The use of minimal pair contrasts (pin/bin, tea/sea, cap/tap), for example, is the key to phonological therapy (Weiner, 1981) and such material can easily be adapted to encompass sound segmentation, rhyming and chunking games for the purpose of speech, reading and spelling developments.

When devising these tasks, therapists need to remind themselves of the multisensory approach and expand the traditional auditory–vocal modality of work. The goal is for the child to recognize the auditory and visual commonalities in the word structure, to experience the articulatory and motor pattern of the word through simultaneous speech production and handwriting, and eventually to move from imitation and copying to spontaneous speech and writing.

In order to accomplish this goal, Bradley (1981) recommends strictly following a series of ordered steps when spelling. The child must propose the word he wants to spell; see it formed by a skilled speller; name it; write it, saying each letter name as he goes; name the word again, and then check that it is written correctly. This procedure is repeated twice. Practice continues for six days with approximately 30 seconds spent on each word. The success of this approach indicates the need for structured and repeated teaching with these children.

READING AND SPELLING RULES

When working directly on reading and spelling rules with the older child it is again important to check what other systems the child is exposed to and provide back up help with this. The Helen Arkell Dyslexia Centre[1] supplies useful literature and materials for therapists, teachers and parents which will help link the child's work across situations.

An invaluable text by Hornsby and Shear (1982) is 'Alpha to Omega'. This is particularly useful for the speech therapists, since it can incorporate colour codes such as the Edith Norrie Letter Case. The programme is divided into three stages, covering a spelling range of 7–15 years, and includes reading, spelling and verbal expression exercises. Advice is also given on handwriting, material and examination technique for the older child (see Hornsby, this volume). Pollock's (1983) 'Signposts to Spelling', with its history of spelling, incorporates humorous cartoons and activities to tackle some of the more tricky English spelling rules.

Recently available is the Aston Portfolio (Aubrey, Eaves, Hicks and Newton) which is based on the Aston Index and gives ideas for the further assessment and teaching of reading (including both visual and auditory skills), spelling, handwriting, comprehension and written expression. It is presented in an easy card index form.

There is already a wealth of teaching materials available with which the speech therapist needs to become familiar. She has a key role in tailoring established schemes to fit *individual* children with persisting speech and language difficulties. This refinement will be based on a full assessment of the child's skills, but will be influenced greatly by chronological age.

[1]The Helen Arkell Dyslexia Centre, 14 Crondace Road, London, SW6

Timing and Type of Intervention

It has been shown that early intervention, focusing on auditory organization skills, plus explicit alphabetic and articulatory work can accelerate reading and spelling progress. Given the results of retrospective studies (Ingram, Mason & Blackburn, 1970; Rutter and Yule, 1973) where junior school aged children with reading problems were found to have had earlier speech and language difficulties, it is likely that the speech therapist will be involved with the child long before he reaches school age and the teacher's expertise. She therefore needs to be able to identify the 'at risk' child and instigate remedial measures early enough to enable the child to have an easier start to school life.

The speech therapist's role in this area would appear to be a continuous one. The children with persisting difficulties may require help and support through and beyond the school years. There is a danger that as intelligibility reaches an acceptable level, the child is discharged from the speech therapist's care only to be left struggling with residual speech difficulties and related spelling problems. The speech therapist may like to consider an advisory role here in order to help the child compensate for articulatory difficulties and liaise with school and home as to appropriate reading and spelling strategies and activities.

'Critical' periods in the learning process, however, need to be considered when dealing with the older child with persisting speech and spelling difficulties. Returning to one of the cases discussed above as an example, L.B., aged 15 years, has had years of phonics training but is functioning below a five-year-level on tests of auditory organization. As he has only one remaining year in school it may be more worthwhile to focus on visual memory training with the emphasis on chunking letter groups rather than to continue on phonics and auditory training. This highlights the importance of individual qualitative assessments as a prerequisite to selecting the most appropriate management strategies. The speech therapist is well equipped to carry out these assessments and has an important role to play in the management of reading and spelling difficulties.

Part 3

Approaches to the Treatment of Reading and Spelling Difficulties

Beve Hornsby

7 A Structured Phonetic/Linguistic Method for Teaching Dyslexics

Teaching the 'Dyslexic'

It is difficult for the competent reader and speller to understand the problems confronting the dyslexic. Proficient readers can decipher unfamiliar words without difficulty. This can frequently be done at the morphemic level because sound 'chunks' have already been learned and internalized. The dyslexic finds the automatic translation from sounds to letters and letters to sounds difficult. He or she has to develop strategies for reading and writing which will avoid the misordering of the letters, produce chunks of sound and ensure that all the syllables in the word are represented. The most successful methods used to date for teaching children with specific learning difficulties concentrate not only on reading and spelling but also on handwriting. In this way spelling concepts are reinforced through visual, auditory and kinaesthetic modalities.

In the U.K. a structured phonetic/linguistic method is used in virtually all centres where dyslexia is taken seriously. Unfortunately the phonic approach is frequently misunderstood. Phonic teaching sometimes involves teaching associations between letter shapes and *single* letter sounds without using the names of the letters at all.

This is a mistake for the following reasons:

1) Teaching single letter sound associations only works when a word's letter/sound relationship is totally regular and the word only has one syllable. For example, the word 'bet' can be sounded out by its single letter sounds /b/ /e/ /t/ whereas 'betting' cannot. One has to use letter names to describe the double 'tt' in the middle and the 'ing' at the end. Similarly with such simple common words such as 'her', 'for', 'car' or 'she', the child needs to know the letter names to be able to say which letters are needed for the vowel sounds at the ends of these words.

2) Many children come to school already knowing the names of the letters and find it confusing to have to call them by something different, i.e. sounds.

3) Letter names are the only things that are constant. Letter sounds change according to the context in which they are used in words.

For example, the letter 'a' has a number of sounds: /æ/ as in 'cat', /ə/ as in 'about', /a/ as in 'banana', and /eɪ/ as in 'aeroplane' and so on. It also has an enormous variety of sounds in vowel digraphs.

Thus, although sounds and sound patterns are essential for reading, names are essential for spelling in order to describe the combinations of letters needed to represent the 44 sounds of English.

It is preferable to have a thorough knowledge of phonetics and linguistics to teach well. However, the talented teacher should find a way to reach the dyslexic child provided a highly structured, systematic approach is adopted, allowing sufficient time for consolidation of newly acquired concepts.

Thorough medical check-ups are essential if there is any reason to suppose that a child has vision, hearing or health problems which need attention before the question of teaching is contemplated. Similarly, psychological investigations are important in order to find out what a child's particular weaknesses are so that his remedial programme can incorporate activities to mitigate them. During the course of a psychological assessment the perceptive clinician will also find out what the child's interests are and what sort of approach is likely to 'switch him on'. No matter what the child's interest, he should be encouraged to read and write about it, even if this means endless comic books! If learning is made dull and boring it will certainly be resisted.

The 'Alpha to Omega' Scheme

Teachers and therapists agree that the key to success with children who have specific learning difficulties is usually a highly structured multi-sensory approach. Here, one particular approach, 'Alpha to Omega' (Hornsby and Shear, 1975), will be outlined in the hope that practising clinicians will be able to adapt this to the individual needs of the child with whom they are working. It is crucial when utilizing this scheme, or a similar one, never to *assume* knowledge of concepts which have not been explicitly taught. Similarly, time should not be wasted teaching concepts which are already established! Teaching should be cumulative, always laying new knowledge on a firm foundation otherwise the advantage of the structure will be lost.

Thus, when following a structured programme such as 'Alpha to Omega', the pupil should be taught logically step by step, beginning with single-letter sounds linked to letter names and letter shapes. In stages, he should progress through simple one syllable words to complex multisyllabic words. To reiterate, as this cannot be stressed enough, the teaching drills should be based on a 'multisensory' technique – one that utilizes the pupil's senses of sight and hearing, as well as involving writing down and reading back what has been written.

Single Letter–Sound Correspondences

The method which 'Alpha to Omega' recommends for teaching letter–sound associations is as follows:

1) The teacher presents the letter on a flashcard with the key picture drawn on the reverse side. It is called a key picture because it unlocks the sound. The pupil should say the letter's name. (See Figure 7.1.)

2) The teacher says the keyword and then the sound of the letter.

3) The pupil repeats the keyword and the sound.

4) The teacher says the sound and then the name.

5) The pupil repeats the sound and gives the name, writing it as he says it (translating the sound he has heard into written letters).

6) The pupil reads what he has written, giving the sound (translating the letters written into sounds that are heard).

7) The pupil writes the letter with the eyes closed to get the feel of the letter (when vision is cut off, other senses such as touch are sharpened).

When the child is reasonably familiar with the names, sounds and shapes of the letters, this drill can be modified to:

1) The pupil runs through the flashcards saying their sounds aloud (the reading process).

2) The teacher then dictates each letter sound in random order for the pupil to say the letter's name and then write it down (the spelling process).

This drill should be repeated with each set of new sound patterns shown on the cards. To accelerate reading skill, cards can be given for reading practice that show more advanced patterns than have yet been reached in spelling. This will also help to familiarize the child with the spelling patterns by the time he is expected to spell them.

The association between single-letter name, sound and shape should be taught first, along with the knowledge that some of these letters are

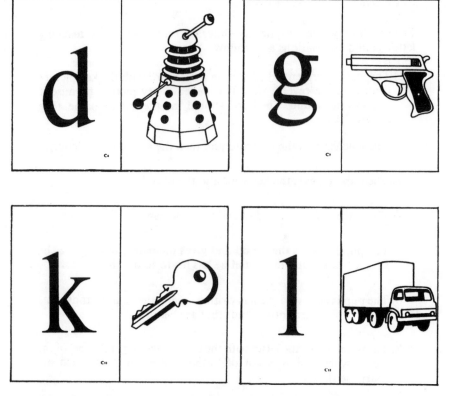

Figure 7.1 Examples of 'Alpha to Omega' flashcards: consonants. (Front and reverse sides shown adjacent to each other)

vowels, which will be needed in every word. The five basic vowels should then be taught including the semi-vowel 'y'. 'Y' is more often a vowel than it is a consonant, since it is only a consonant at the beginning of words. Everywhere else in a word, 'y' is a vowel and is used instead of 'i' because no English words end in 'i'. When 'y' is a vowel it has the same sounds as 'i', either long as in 'by', or short as in 'gypsy'. The vowels have the key picture on the front along with the letter, as the child needs this visual mnemonic when choosing which vowel to use. (See Figure 7.2.)

You will notice that the letters on the flashcards are all in print. However, when the child writes the letter he may write it in script. It is difficult to lay down any hard and fast rules about handwriting, but it is essential that children should be taught *how* to form letters correctly and where each letter should start. Handwriting, like spelling, can so easily be taught in a structured manner (Alston and Taylor, 1984; see also Augur, this volume).

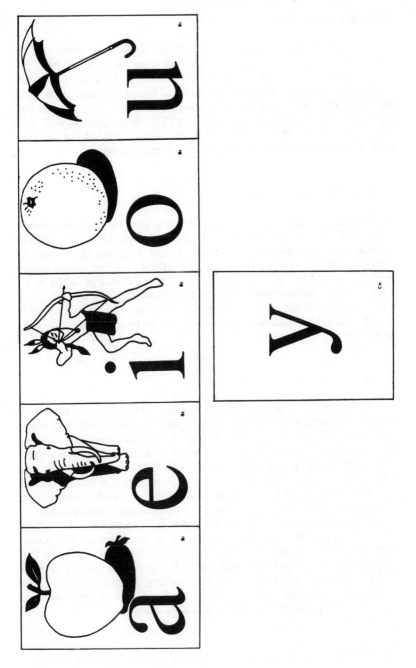

Figure 7.2 Flashcards from 'Alpha to Omega': vowels. (These cards should be in front of child during work on vowel discrimination)

Open and Closed Syllables

The concept of the open and closed syllable needs to be explained to children for them to understand that 'go' does not need to be spelt 'gow'. Since there is not a consonant on the end of the word, the vowel sounds like its name. If the syllable is closed by a consonant, as in 'got' and 'god' the vowel then becomes short. (This concept is crucial for more advanced work upon spelling rules.) The books 'Spellbound' and 'The Spell of Words' by Elsie Rak are recommended for further explanation of the concept of open and closed syllables.

Consonant Blends and Digraphs

Many pupils will have to be introduced to the 'chunking' of consonants and vowels and taught that certain combinations of letters are needed to make certain sounds. For example, 's' and 'h' giving /ʃ/, 'c' and 'h' giving /tʃ/, and 't' and 'h' producing either /ð/, the hard or voiced sound as in the word 'the', or /θ/, the soft or voiceless sound as in the word 'thin'. Then come the consonant blends, such as 'br', 'pl', 'spr' and after these the vowel/consonant digraphs like 'er', 'or', 'ar' and so on. It is obvious that this is necessry if 44 sounds are to be represented by only 26 letters.

'Hierarchical' Letter Sound Rules

Soon after the child has mastered the consonant digraphs, he should be taught that certain letters influence or modify the vowels that come after them. The letter 'w', for example, changes the sound of most of the vowels that follow it. Hence 'was' is not spelt 'wos', 'war' is not spelt 'wor' and 'worm' is not spelt 'werm'. A difficult concept such as this must be introduced with the help of many mnemonics, illustrations and so forth. Another difficult concept which requires careful explanation is that some consonants have more than one sound. For example, 'c' and 'g' both have this characteristic. When followed by 'e', 'i' or 'y', 'c' sounds like /s/ as in 'city', or 'g' sounds like /dʒ/ as in 'gentle'. Of course, there are some extremely common words which do not adhere to this rule, such as 'get,' 'girl' and 'gift' but it is regularly followed in most words and helps with reading as well as spelling. Useful workbooks for reinforcing these concepts are 'Space to Spell' and 'More Space to Spell' by Shear, Targett and Raines (1977).

Final Syllables

Gradually the complete range of spelling patterns and rules should be covered, culminating in the final syllables 'tion', 'sion', 'cian', 'tial', 'cious', 'cient', 'tient', 'cial' and so on. The English language contains many such oddities and irregularities which have to be explained to the dyslexic.

It is perhaps now obvious why a detailed knowledge of phonetics is desirable if a phonetic approach is to be taught successfully. Eventually, the question of stress in multisyllable words will need working on, since this dictates whether or not consonants are doubled in spelling. These, and other advanced concepts, are described in the final stage of 'Alpha to Omega'.

From Words to Sentences

As Klein's chapter points out, many dyslexics find it hard to form sentences using the words they have learnt. Whilst working upon spelling patterns and concepts it is therefore advisable for the teacher to pay attention to the way in which the child structures his language. Dyslexics should be introduced by dictation to sentence formation in its simplest form in the early stages. Asking a child to write in simple, active, affirmative, declarative sentences (SAAD) is advantageous as it reduces memory load and encourages organization in writing. Examples of SAADs given in 'Alpha to Omega' include:

(A) The man ran to the red van.

(B) A black cat jumped on the table.

Note, however, that the phonetic content of sentences must be matched to the pupil's level of spelling competence. Sentence (A) could be introduced at an early stage because it contains phonetically regular words, whereas sentence (B) features many spelling and sound patterns that may not have been taught. For instance:

a) The consonant blend 'bl' at the beginning of the word 'black'.

b) The 'ck' ending which is only used in one-syllable words after a short vowel.

c) The spelling of the regular past tense 'ed', which never sounds like /ɛd/.

d) The final syllable 'ble' which has a sound similar to 'bull' in the word 'table'.

The method used for dictating sentences is again based on the multisensory technique, involving the pupil in listening, speaking, writing, seeing and reading.

1) Dictate the whole sentence as you would normally say it.

2) Ask the pupil to repeat it aloud.

3) Dictate it again, isolating each word and speaking very clearly so that the words are not heard running together in strings, but separated as they will be written down.

4) The pupil writes the sentence, saying it clearly as he writes it. (He is now making the translation from spoken to written language for himself.)

5) Ask the pupil to read aloud what he has written.

6) Suggest final corrections if the pupil fails to discover them for himself. Try not to tell him what he should have written; rather lead him to discover for himself by providing appropriate clues and encourage him to make double checking of all his work second nature.

7) Finally, ask the pupil to read the sentence with expression as though it were being spoken.

This method also increases the child's memory for sentences, since you start with short sentences and progress to increasingly longer ones. The complexity of transformations from SAAD to other sentence forms is also structured and cumulative, being taught in the following order:

1) The SAAD sentence – 'A rat is a pet'.

2) The question – but only at the simple reversal of verb level, 'Is a rat a pet?' More difficult types of question structure should only be introduced later on; for example, the tag question. This can either be a negative tag to a positive statement: 'It is a nice day, isn't it?', or a positive tag to a negative statement: 'It isn't a nice day, is it?'.

3) The negative, but again only at the simple level, e.g. 'A rat is not a pet'. Note that the negative can be difficult both to understand and produce. A sentence like 'Twenty-one is not an even number' may well cause confusion.

4) The compound sentence, consisting of more than one principle clause, as in: 'That cat can sit on my lap, but that dog cannot'.

5) The negative question, with or without tags. For instance 'It isn't fun at school, is it?'

6) The complex sentence, consisting of a principle clause and one or more subordinate clauses, as in: 'The man, who wore a leather coat, hit the dog'.

7) Cause and effect: 'I wanted to marry him, but I could not stand his mother'.

8) The passive: 'The dog was beaten by the man in the leather coat'.

9) The negative passive: 'The dog was not beaten by the man in the leather coat'.

As mentioned in the drill for dictating of sentences, it must be made clear to the dyslexic that words are not written as they are spoken. The flow of sound in running speech has to be broken up into isolated words to avoid the confusions that were evidently in the mind of the 14-year-old who wrote 'I came to school smorning'. It is necessary to explain that it could have been that morning, the other morning, yesterday morning, tomorrow morning, as well as this morning! The dyslexic can only learn to break up the verbal strings of speech correctly by writing practice using full sentences.

Case Studies

The simplest way of illustrating how to begin to teach is to take a series of children who have been assessed and from these assessments, outline a possible teaching programme. In a structured linguistic programme such as 'Alpha to Omega', the natural progression needs to be followed, but teachers will be called upon to help people of all ages and at all levels of literacy competence and of intellectual ability. It is necessary, therefore, to be able to adapt the recognized structure (which must be very familiar to the teacher or therapist) to accommodate the individual needs and interests of every person referred.

Case 1 David

The first child we will discuss is David, a boy who was referred at an early age, 6 years 7 months, but whose poor progress with reading and spelling was of concern, given his superior I.Q. (Verbal I.Q. 125, Performance I.Q. 115, Full Scale I.Q. 122.)

On the Neale Analysis of Reading Ability the text is as follows:

'A black cat came to my house. She put her kitten by the door. Then she went away. Now I have her baby for a pet.'

David read as follows:

'A blue cat come to my home. .... by the ..... Ho I live blue blue .. a .....'

David knew the names of the letters and most of the sounds but he had not yet been able to associate the two. When presented with

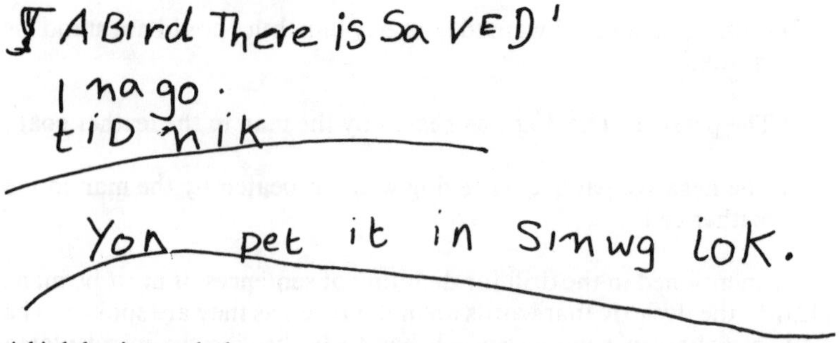

ʃ A Bird There is Sa VE D '

I na go .

t i D n i k

Yon pet it in Sinwg lok.

A bird that is squashed

— —

Dried milk

You put it in someone's drink

Figure 7.3 Free writing from David, aged 6 years 7 months, Verbal I.Q. 123

phonetically regular words for reading he was at a loss because he had no idea of how to work them out by their sounds. He did not yet know the letters and sounds of the vowels. On the Midland Spelling Scale David had a spelling age of less than 5 years. His errors included 'mai' for 'may', 'dod' for 'did', 'goe' for 'grow'. He could write his first name, but not his surname. Not surprisingly, David's attempt to write a story was pitiful (Figure. 7.3) and despite the fact that he had a good grasp of spoken language, he could not write a comprehensible sentence. Indeed, it will be some time before his written vocabulary will permit him to write stories on his own.

It is clear that David is virtually a 'nonstarter'. He requires teaching from first principles using the 'Alpha to Omega' scheme. Initially a small sample of consonants might be introduced for reading and for writing. Consonants which can be confused neither visually nor phonologically should be chosen (for example n, t, b, s, g). David should aim to give the names and the sounds of these consonants automatically on confrontation and to write them to dictation. With the introduction of just two vowels (again nonconfusable ones such as 'a' and 'i'), many simple words can be built (bat, sat, tin, sin, bin, bit, big), plural – s can be demonstrated and soon short sentences can be written to dictation, e.g. 'The bat sat in the bin'.

Case 2 Noel

Whether or not children should be taught individually is a moot point. There are undoubtedly advantages of teaching a child with a peer in that they may be able to help each other in a sensitive and supportive manner. Nonetheless, when teaching in groups it is crucial to make the teaching programme individualized.

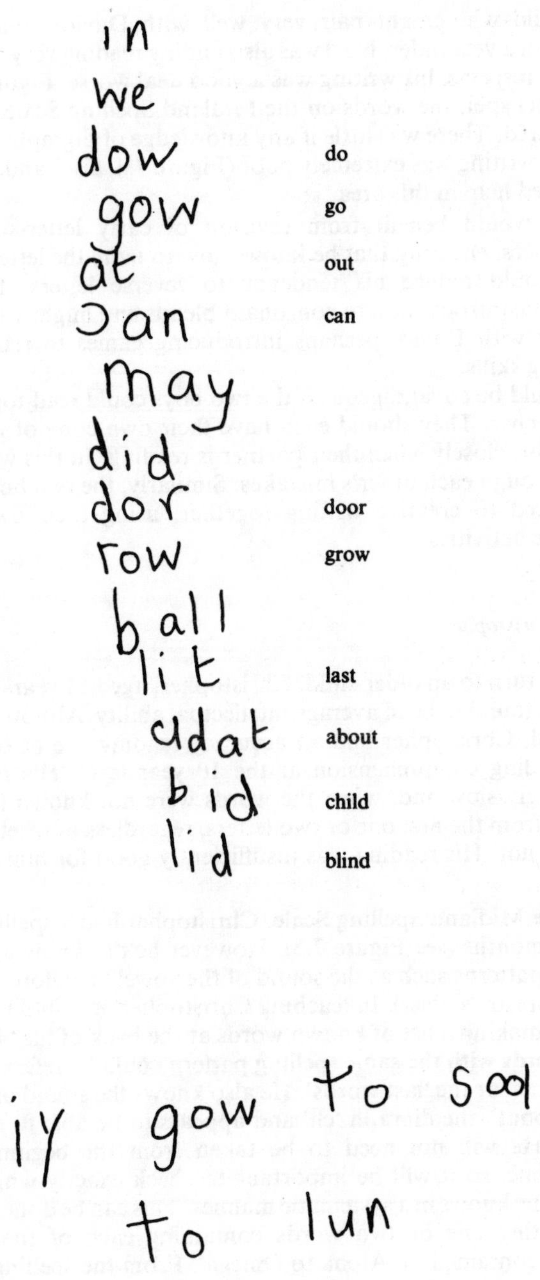

in
we
dow   do
gow   go
at   out
ɔan   can
may
did
dor   door
row   grow
ball
lit   last
udat   about
bid   child
lid   blind

iy gow to sool to lun

I go to school to learn

Figure 7.4 Spelling and free writing produced by Noel, aged 8 years, Verbal I.Q. 107

A child who might pair very well with David would be Noel. Although a year older, Noel was also finding reading very difficult and, in some respects, his writing was a good deal worse. Figure 7.4 shows how Noel spelt the words on the Midland Spelling Scale. Some were misordered. There was little if any knowledge of digraphs and blends. His free writing was extremely poor (Figure 7.4, also) and, like David, he needed help in this area.

Noel would benefit from revision of early letter-sound correspondences, ensuring that he knows how to *write* the letters properly. This should reduce his tendency to reverse letters. He requires systematic introduction to consonant blends and might work on these together with David, perhaps introducing games to reinforce their emerging skills.

It would be advantageous if the two boys could read together, with their teacher. They should each have their own copy of the text and follow this closely when their partner is reading. In this way they can learn through each other's mistakes. Similarly, the two boys might be introduced to creative writing together, using their own ideas to structure activities.

Case 3 Christopher

Now we turn to an older child, Christopher, aged 11 years 10 months, who was found to be of average intellectual ability. Although nearly 12 years old, Christopher had an accuracy reading age of only 9 years with reading comprehension at the 10 year level. His reading was agonizingly slow and, when the words were not known by sight, he guessed from the first one or two letters, regardless of whether it made sense or not. His reading was insufficiently good for him to read for pleasure.

On the Midland Spelling Scale, Christopher had a spelling age of 7 years 9 months (see Figure 7.5). However he did know a number of spelling patterns such as the sound of the vowel 'a' before an 'l' (ball), and before an 's' (last). In teaching Christopher, it would be helpful to start by making a list of known words at the back of his book so that other words with the same spelling pattern could be referred to as the 'ball words' or the 'last words'. He also knows the sound of 'ou' in the word 'about', the digraph 'ch' and appears to be able to manage the blends. He will not need to be taken from the beginning of the programme, so it will be important to check exactly which spelling patterns he knows in a systematic manner. This can be done most easily by dictating one or two words containing each of the individual patterns contained in 'Alpha to Omega'. From the spelling test alone we know that he has not grasped the spelling patterns 'oi' or 'igh'. These could be possible starting points.

Christopher also desperately needs help with syllabification. His spellings of family (famel) and punishment (punshmet) indicate his

ball
last
about
child
blind

famel	family
ponr	point
perhas	perhaps
pertecton	protection
mertoin	motion
frited	frighten
punshmet	punishment
continu	continue
poshon	portion
constuted	construct

I got the computer on chrismus i did
not no waht to do wiht it so i lete
my dad fixy it up so I colud do
thins with it we had a tape.
now we got a disdrip it can do
eney think it ~~the so~~ loads games in 3 secony

Figure 7.5 Spelling and free writing produced by Christopher, aged 11 years 10 months

tendency to omit syllables when writing words. It is interesting that the final syllable 'tion' has been partly mastered but, without good sequencing skills, words with this ending cannot be spelled accurately. Christopher's spelling problem is even more apparent during free writing. When he has to concentrate upon the content of his work, he is all the more prone to misorder letters and to omit consonants from blends. (See Figure 7.5.) Christopher needs to be encouraged to sound out phonemic segments when writing them. In addition, he would benefit from some explanation of the sound structure of polysyllabic words. His pronunciation of specific words needs sharpening, particularly so that he can write words like 'disc-drive' and 'Christmas'.

With a step-by-step approach, it should be possible to improve Christopher's spelling skills dramatically. His passion for computers might be usefully employed by the innovative teacher and possibly software packages of games might be carefully selected to reinforce specific spelling concepts.

An unfortunate consequence of Christopher's reading disability has been that, although he had a very good spoken vocabulary when young, this has deteriorated. It will be important for his teacher to help him to extend his knowledge and use of words. After he has finished reading a passage, it would be a good idea to discuss the meaning of some of the words and explore other meanings the same words might have. Words that appeal to Christopher could then be written in a personal dictionary with their definitions. He should be encouraged to use them as often as possible so that they become automatic enough to be used in free writing and examinations. Given the stage of reading which Christopher has reached, this seems to be the most appropriate way to proceed, together with the structured assistance with spelling skills already outlined.

Case 4 Mary

Finally, we turn to a young adult, Mary, aged 17 years 9 months. Mary was originally diagnosed dyslexic when she was seven, but she has received little structured assistance on account of being away at boarding school. She is an intelligent girl (Full Scale WAIS I.Q. = 118) who has overcome her reading difficulties but she has a persistent spelling problem. She scored at the 16th percentile on the Wide Range Achievement Test and, as her free writing shows (see Figure 7.6), she still misorders letters in words, leaves out syllables, and confuses 'p', 'd' and 'b'.

It would be possible with Mary to start by checking her knowledge of the individual spelling patterns comprising 'Alpha to Omega'. Evidently she has already mastered the basic spelling patterns and concepts of the earlier stages and furthermore, she has much advanced orthographic knowledge. A more pragmatic approach would be to look at the written work which she is doing for college and to work on those spelling patterns that are shaky. Relevant portions of 'Alpha to Omega' could then be selected. For instance, in her free writing, Mary wrote 'year' correctly once but as 'yare' on another occasion. This error might lead to a lesson on words containing 'ear', pronounced /ɪə/. A list of such words (ear, fear, near, spear and so on), plus sentences for dictation, is included in the programme. Mary might also revise the 'soft c' rule, if indeed she knows it at all. Her spellings of choice (chose) and decide (deside) suggest she is uncertain of its use.

It goes without saying that punctuation and syntax need attention and Mary needs to develop an effective strategy for checking her own work through. Together with her teacher she should work explicitly on the specialized vocabulary which she needs for her course. In the long

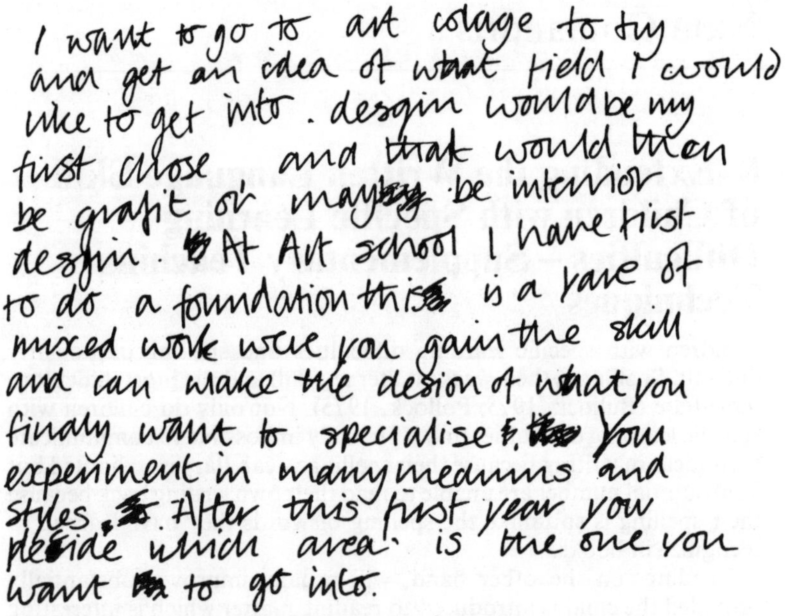

I want to go to art colage to try
and get an idea of what field I would
like to get into. desgin would be my
first close and that would then
be grafit or maybe be interior
desgin. At Art school I have first
to do a foundation this is a yare of
mixed work were you gain the skill
and can make the desion of what you
finaly want to specialise. You
experiment in many mediums and
styles. After this first year you
decide which area is the one you
want to go into.

Figure 7.6 Free writing from Mary, aged 17 years, Verbal I.Q. 125

term, she might be encouraged to learn to type; this would no doubt
help her with letter order and to consolidate new spellings. Also it
would improve the presentation of her work which is rather difficult to
read due to her italic handwriting.

The main point of the above cases has been to show that 'Alpha to
Omega', although a highly structured phonetic/linguistic programme,
is an extremely flexible one which the skilled teacher can adapt to the
needs of the individual pupil. The great advantage of the method is that
it can form the backbone of a treatment programme whilst still
allowing the teacher a free rein to introduce other games and activities
which may be particularly helpful to the person with whom they are
working. It should not need restating that to capture the interest of the
pupil is of enormous consequence. Once this has been done, a
systematic, cumulative approach can be adopted within which the
child *cannot* fail. Every success will breed greater motivation and there
will be a noticeable effect, not only upon educational progress but also
upon morale.

Nata Goulandris

8 Extending the Written Language Skill of Children with Specific Learning Difficulties – Supplementary Teaching Techniques

Children with specific learning difficulties find spelling particularly difficult. Spelling is their weakest literacy skill and the most difficult to remediate (Bullock, 1975; Pollock, 1975). Not only do children with specific learning difficulties find it virtually impossible to communicate their ideas in writing because their spelling vocabulary is so limited but a substantial number are unable to read their own writing back because their spelling is so unlike the spelling of words they have learned to recognize in books.

Reading, on the other hand, will usually improve substantially provided the child is introduced to reading matter which is interesting to him and which is well within his reading ability. Once enjoyable reading material is found, a combination of reading for meaning supported by phonic and 'look and say' methods almost always results in improved reading skill.

The reason that reading is so much easier to remediate than spelling is that reading requires only partial visual cues (Frith and Frith, 1980). Even the beginner reader has a wealth of knowledge about the world and the events he is reading about. He can therefore predict with relative accuracy the types of words he might encounter, considering the situation of the characters in the story he is reading. By five, the infant school child also has good command of the English language and he can use semantic, syntactic and phonological cues to facilitate reading performance (Smith, 1971; LaBerge and Samuels, 1974).

In contrast, spelling requires full cues. In order to write a word a child needs to recall all the letters, in their correct order. To do this the child must either refer to a perfect visual image or to an exact orthographic representation of the word. Alternatively, he will be forced to sound out the word and use letter–sound correspondence rules (always a precarious approach). In other words, whereas the child only needs to recognize words when reading, he must recall each one of the requisite letters when spelling. So spelling is a much more exacting process than reading.

A further difference between reading and spelling is that there are fewer ways in which a given grapheme can be pronounced (reading) than there are ways in which a phoneme can be written (spelling) (Cronnell, 1978). English orthography permits several alternative graphemes for the same phoneme. The sound /ō/ can be spelled 'o' as in

134

'only', 'oa' as in 'boat', 'oe' as in 'toe', 'ow' as in 'throw' and 'ough' as in 'though'.

Similarly, the sound /k/ can be spelled with a 'c' as in 'cat', 'k' as in 'kitten', 'ck' as in 'duck', 'ch' as in 'Christmas' and 'que' as in 'unique'. Clearly, a phonological strategy on its own will not help the speller decide which of these plausible alternatives to select. On the other hand, an orthographic strategy would enable the speller to do so without recourse to phonology.

The use of an orthographic strategy in spelling implies that the speller can access an internal representation of the word which specifies both the requisite letters and their correct order. (See Snowling, this volume.) It is not clear how this memory representation is coded. Some people say that they can evoke visual images of the words which they know. Others cannot do this but may represent spelling knowledge in alphabetic, syllabic or morphemic form.

Finally, it is generally agreed that skilled spelling is an automatic motor skill which requires no thought but flows smoothly and inevitably until the required word is formed (Schonell, 1942; Peters, 1967). It is this automatic skill which we seek to foster in our pupils.

The traditional belief that accurate spelling is primarily acquired by rote learning has recently fallen from favour. However, several researchers have concluded that the good speller is inclined to examine words closely (Frith, 1980) and to note similarities with other familiar words (Peters, 1967). To this extent spelling knowledge is dependent upon specific reading experiences.

The developmental theories of spelling proposed amongst others by Read (1980), Henderson (1980) and Beers (1980) contend that the acquisition of spelling ability parallels the acquisition of language. In both cases children form hypotheses, use over-generalizations and gradually refine these generalizations to incorporate linguistic exceptions. Both the precocious pre-school child who is often not reading yet and the beginning speller who has just commenced school are able to encode by developing theories about English orthography. They begin by constructing theories about the short vowels and the consonants while totally ignoring long vowels. Later, they become aware of the differences between long and short vowels and they begin to use long vowel markers in their spelling. Children proceed from the assumption that written language is based exclusively on speech sounds to an understanding of the complex interrelationship between the phonological, the morphemic and the etymological levels of English orthography.

If this process seems surprisingly complex for a young child, it is well to remember that he has already acquired remarkable verbal ability at a much younger age precisely through the process of making hypotheses and generalizations and revising them when necessary.

Gradually, the beginning speller acquires an unconscious understanding of the rules underlying English spelling. He acquires what Margaret Peters (1970) calls an understanding of 'serial probability'.

He knows what looks right. He has expectations and can make predictions. He is able to construct plausible approximations for unknown words and he is able to use these expectations to help him remember unexpected spellings. In short, he has not learned a diverse assortment of spellings but has been able to construct a basic overview of the patterns of English spelling.

It is just such an overview which the child with specific learning difficulties lacks and it is generally recognized that specific teaching will be required to relay this knowledge to those children who have been unable to abstract it for themselves.

A Structured Cumulative Approach

As Hornsby (this volume) makes clear, a structured cumulative approach is a systematic teaching course which increases in difficulty in small progressive steps. This gradual and cumulative acquisition of knowledge ensures success and bolsters the child's self-confidence and sense of accomplishment. At the same time the number of errors is reduced to a minimum since a pupil is only expected to know the material he has already been taught. Multisensory learning is achieved by the simultaneous use of all the senses normally required for written language skills: visual, auditory, tactile–kinaesthetic and oral–kinaesthetic. Multisensory learning enables a child to learn by using his intact sensory channels while at the same time making use of his weaker channels. Because the child is learning through four interrelated sensory pathways, learning is more successful and inadequate modalities are bypassed. Although there is as yet no research to prove that the structured cumulative phonic approach is more efficient than other possible alternative methods, most teachers who use it to provide a core structure find it extremely effective.

The reasons why a cumulative, structured, multisensory, phonic programme is particularly successful for children with specific learning difficulties can be easily understood. Dyslexic children have difficulty with certain phonological tasks such as rhyming and phonemic segmentation (Bradley and Bryant, 1978). They are, therefore, unable to acquire the implicit understanding of phoneme–grapheme relationships which the normal child acquires in the course of normal spelling and reading acquisition (Snowling, 1980). By providing these children with the most rudimentary knowledge of phoneme–grapheme relationships using all modalities, we enable these poor readers and spellers to

1) learn to use first letter cues

2) begin to chunk groups of letters which frequently occur together in the English language such as 'oa', 'ing', 'ight', etc

3) acquire sufficient skill to use phonology for their initial spelling attempts – a strategy which many normal pre-school children adopt in their first attempts to capture spoken language on paper.

Several approaches of the type outlined above are currently in use in the U.K. These include 'Alpha to Omega' by Hornsby and Shear (1976); 'Dyslexia: A Language Teaching Course for Teachers and Learners' by Hickey, and 'Diagnosis in the Classroom' by Cotterell. All begin by teaching simple one to one phoneme–grapheme correspondence rules so that children can quickly learn to build up simple regular words. The children are taught the name and sound of each letter, and how to write it. Words are presented in groups which are both visually and phonologically similar. For example, a group of words containing the sound /ar/ such as 'car', 'far', 'lard', 'farm', 'scarf' and 'hard' is presented all at the same time. Dictation is used to encourage a child to construct the spelling of regular words. The children are also introduced to irregular words and they are shown that these will require other types of learning technique.

Structured, phonic methods initially begin with a strong emphasis on phonological spelling but as the children progress the emphasis shifts towards an understanding of morphology, in particular the use of prefixes and suffixes, and more stress is placed on the use of visual memory. (See Hornsby, this volume, for further discussion.)

In this chapter some procedures which complement but do not replace the use of a structured cumulative approach will be described and some alternative methods for teaching children with visuo–orthographic difficulties will be suggested.

'Whole Word' Learning Techniques

In 1943, Fernald introduced 'whole word' methods of learning spelling for children with severe reading and spelling problems. She advocated the use of tracing. The child is asked which word he wants to learn and this word is written in large cursive letters on a card. The teacher pronounces the word distinctly and the child is requested to repeat it. The child is then required to trace over the word with his finger while pronouncing each syllable as he traces it. When the child believes that he has learned to spell the word he tries to write it from memory. If he succeeds, he writes it from memory again. If the word is incorrect he begins the finger tracing again until he feels ready to attempt the word from memory once more.

This kinaesthetic method relies on the child learning to reproduce exact, automatic, spelling motor movements and so bypasses phonological intervention. It is, therefore, frequently recommended as the best method for teaching sight words or for teaching children whose phonological deficits are so great that phonological methods are counter-productive. It does, however, have the disadvantage of being extremely boring and after the initial interest children find it increasingly difficult to concentrate on the tracing, with a resultant loss of benefit. It therefore seems wise to transfer to less monotonous 'whole word' methods as soon as it is thought appropriate.

Bradley's (1981) Simultaneous Oral Spelling method is a possible alternative. The word is written for the child or constructed with plastic letters. The child is asked to say the word, then writes the word in cursive script, naming each letter as he writes it. Finally, the child checks to see if the word is correct and repeats the spelling sequence once more.

Peters' (1967, 1970) technique of LOOK (i.e. study), COVER, WRITE, CHECK is a valuable method for teaching children to examine and learn words. The child is required to study the word until he feels he knows it, to cover the correct version, to attempt the spelling and then to check his spelling against the correct version. For this method to be successful with children with specific learning difficulties, the teacher should ask the child to verbalize the difference between the word he has written and the correct version. Children often prefer simply to have another 'go' without taking the time to understand and specify verbally exactly where the error lay. This method is used by many classroom teachers and it may already be familiar to the child.

Bradley's simultaneous oral spelling combines articulating the names of the letters with writing the word simultaneously. Her method differs from Peters' in that children are asked to copy the word as part of the learning process before they attempt to write it from memory. In empirical research using children with severe reading and spelling problems (Bradley, 1981) this method was found significantly superior four weeks after teaching than when spelling was (1) not taught; (2) taught by asking the child to say the names of the letters without writing the word and (3) taught by asking the child to repeat the name of the word only as he wrote the word. Although the second and the third methods were superior to the untaught condition, the words learned using the simultaneous oral spelling method were recalled better.

Torbe (1977) essentially agrees with Peters' LOOK, COVER WRITE, CHECK method but he also suggests that the teacher should pronounce the word first and the child should say the word as he studies it. This seems wise, as some children forget which word they're learning even while they are learning it!

In addition Torbe recommends pointing out any difficult or unexpected parts of the word. There is substantial disagreement between authors on this point. Some believe that underlining a difficult part of the word breaks up the continuity of the word and makes it more difficult for the child to learn it. Others feel that if a child is forewarned about the unexpected portion he will make fewer errors. From experience it seems best simply to present the word at the outset but to indicate tricky sections if the child consistently fails to recall that part of the word. Frequently children make errors in totally unexpected portions of the word so it is often not really constructive to try and anticipate their errors.

The selection of the 'whole word' technique most suited to a particular individual is made by trial and error. Begin first with the

LOOK, COVER, WRITE, CHECK method. It will be quite clear if this is not appropriate for this child. He will simply tell you he's learned the word while at the same time being quite unable to write the word from memory. Bradley's Simultaneous Oral Spelling technique can then be presented. If this too proves ineffective, tracing should be used. As a rule of thumb, the less the child knows about letters and their sounds, the more kinaesthetic the whole word method required. As the child becomes more proficient in reading and spelling, he will become more efficient at learning the word visually and will require less kinaesthetic support.

Mnemonics

Although some teachers believe that mnemonics simply require the child to learn irrelevant additional information, poor spellers (especially those with weak visual memories) find them extremely useful for recalling orthographic information. Mnemonics can be pictorial, such as those shown in Figure 8.1.

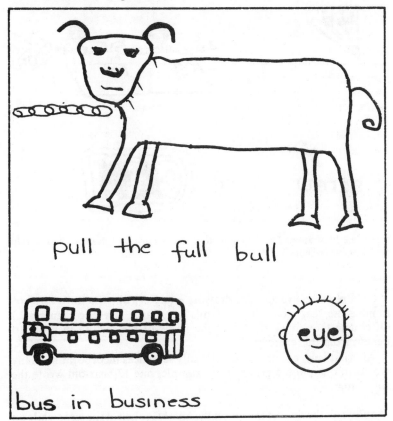

Figure 8.1 Examples of some useful mnemonics

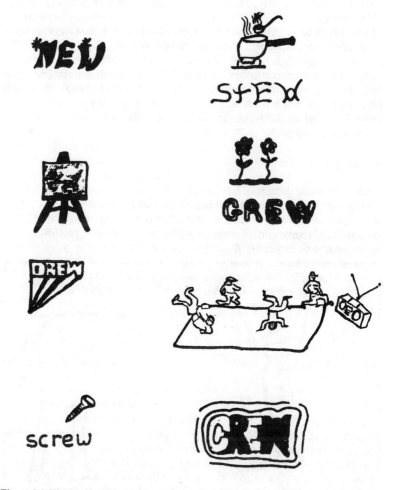

Figure 8.2 Illustrations for spelling pattern 'ew'. Drawn by a dyslexic child to help him learn the spellings

Children who are good at drawing enjoy drawing pictures of word families, i.e. 'car', 'bar', 'jar', 'farm', 'tar', 'lard', etc. (See Figure 8.2.) Of course they must also write the name of the picture in order to benefit from this exercise.

Alternatively, children can write silly sentences incorporating many words in one phonic group. For example, one 12-year-old wrote the following:

'At *night*, in the *light* of the moon the *knight* looked at the *sight* while on his *right* a man got a *fright* while in *flight*.'

He even managed to illustrate every word!

For 'ur' he produced:

'The man m*ur*dered the c*ur*ly haired n*ur*se for her p*ur*se in the ch*ur*ch. He b*ur*nt the ch*ur*ch and went home and ate a t*ur*key and some t*ur*nips. All this happened on Sat*ur*day, not Th*ur*sday.'

Some children use silly sentences to help them remember each letter in a dreaded sight word. For example, 'what' can be recalled as 'We have a tiger.' Although this type of mnemonic appears slightly far-fetched, some children with specific learning difficulties report that this is the only way they can remember some of the words they find particularly difficult.

Although all teachers have some classical mnemonics which are rarely forgotten by their pupils (see Pollock, 1975, for some excellent examples), in general it is preferable for children to construct their own. Presumably, constructing mnemonics makes children examine words more carefully than they normally do and consequently results in a better orthographic representation.

Proof-reading

Proof-reading is probably one of the least taught spelling skills. Unlike reading, proof-reading requires close attention to graphemes. The difficulty is that most children have a tendency to reread their own writing quickly and since they know what they intended to convey they are rarely able to find any spelling errors. Poor readers and spellers are even more likely to find it difficult to notice errors since their internal representations of words are shaky. It is really imperative, therefore, to give instruction in proof-reading. Once a child is able to correct his own spelling it is possible to consider that he is actually becoming a 'speller'.

Personke and Yee (1971) found that boys who had been taught to proof-read, to underline dubious spellings and to use techniques for finding unknown words in the dictionary made significantly fewer errors than controls who had not been taught these techniques.

The teacher can begin proof-reading instruction by underlining errors which she is certain that the pupil can correct and asking him to find them. If the teacher is judicious in her selection the pupil will be able to correct all the words with little difficulty. Often he actually knows how to spell the word but as he was concentrating on creative writing, he was too engrossed in the story to pay attention to the spelling.

It has been found that children with specific learning difficulties make many more errors than normal children who are matched for spelling age (Thomson, 1982). This would suggest that these children have more difficulty concentrating on dual tasks than younger normal children. Therefore, they will require not only basic spelling instruction but also concentrated instruction on spelling in the context of their creative writing.

Once a child becomes adept at finding mistakes which have been pointed out to him, he should be encouraged to question his spelling as he writes. He can, for example, underline words which he feels may be incorrect. Upon completion of the writing he may well be able to supply the correct spelling. If not, he can either check these words in his own personal dictionary, in a normal dictionary or with the teacher. This self questioning is vital for the attainment of correct spelling.

Finally, the teaching of proof-reading must also incorporate dictionary work so that the child can look up words if he is uncertain how to spell them. When a child is able to recite the alphabet correctly, to say which letter precedes or follows a letter, he can begin dictionary work.

The first step requires the introduction of the 'dictionary quartiles' (or quarters of the dictionary). These are A–D, E–M, M–R and S–Z. The child should begin by arranging a wooden alphabet into quartiles so that he has much practice in deciding in which quartile he will find each letter. When the child is familiar with the quartiles and is able to find initial letters without difficulty he can begin building words with different initial letters and then words with similar initial clusters. This type of practice will enable him to understand the alphabetical precedence of one letter over other letters in the same position in the word. Next he will need practice with the dictionary itself, learning to find the correct quartile quickly and accurately.

The dictionary work necessary for proof-reading must be accompanied by thorough grounding in phonological possibilities and order of precedence. To return to the example of the sound /k/, the order of precedence according to frequency of occurrence in the English written language is 'c', 'k', 'ck', 'ch' and 'que'. It is almost impossible to look up a word in the dictionary without this knowledge. A chart of the common vowel and consonant graphemes in use for each phoneme and their order of precedence is helpful for children who do not know this information well.

Games

Spelling games cannot actually teach spelling since this requires conscious attention to the internal form of the words. However, spelling games are useful for reinforcing new spelling rules or spelling patterns or assessing whether old ones are still recalled.

There are many excellent phonic crosswords now available. Picture crosswords are particularly useful because the pupil does not need a high level of reading skill in order to complete them. However, care must be taken when selecting crosswords as some use inappropriately difficult words with elementary letter strings. For example, a child who is learning 'ar' will be able to construct 'car', 'far', 'bar', 'star', but may not yet be able to spell 'farmer' or 'larder' if he has not been introduced to the 'er' spelling. At a later stage, however, these words could provide revision for both letter strings.

A variety of commercial 'snap' and 'rummy' games exist. For example, Phonic Rummy is an American version which consists of several packs graded in order of phonic difficulty. These are highly recommended for reinforcing a child's knowledge of word families.

However, it is relatively easy for teachers to make their own versions. The words included can then be adapted to the child's needs or the particular phonic approach the teacher is using. Useful permutations can include words with the same beginning sounds, final sounds, blends, vowels, identical words (i.e. 'was', 'was') or words which belong to the same phonic group (house, mouse). Morphemes can also be used so that words can be grouped according to their prefixes, suffixes or root words.

A more sophisticated classification game is suggested by Zutel (1980) and Gillet and Kita (1980) and is called 'Word Sorts'. Initially, children are presented with picture cards and asked to sort the pictures into categories, for example fruit and vegetables. Once the children have understood the principle of classification they are given cards of words which are in their reading vocabulary and asked to sort them according to teacher-directed categories such as similarities of phonic elements, vowels, spelling patterns, number of syllables, etc. As the children become more skilled they are asked to determine their own criteria. Children can then play 'Rummy', 'Snap', 'Old Maid' or 'Fish' according to the classification selected. An alternative version requires a group of children to guess what classification one of their members is using. Word Sorts not only encourages children to examine words from different perspectives but it also permits the teacher to monitor the child's level of awareness of words structure.

Edith Norrie Letter Case

The Edith Norrie Letter Case is especially helpful for children with phonological difficulties. The letter case is a box which is divided into compartments each containing one letter or consonant digraph. The letters are not grouped alphabetically but according to the place of articulation of the sound most frequently associated with the letter. For example, letters whose sounds are formed with the lips such as 'm', 'b', 'v', 'p', 'w', 'f', 'wh' are all in the left-hand section of the box. In addition, voiced consonants are printed in green, unvoiced consonants in black and vowels in red. This is very useful for children who frequently confuse voiced and unvoiced sounds.

When the child attempts to spell a word using the letter case he is obliged to work out how he makes the sound in his mouth. The increased awareness of speech sounds and of the relationship between phonemes and graphemes is very beneficial to children who have previously found it very difficult to associate a phoneme with the correct grapheme(s).

Many children also enjoy constructing a word without committing it to paper. They feel it is easier to try different versions and see which one looks correct. They also find that the red vowels help them to see if they have included a vowel in each word or in each syllable.

'Language Experience' Approach

The 'language experience' approach uses the child's own stories as reading material. It is particularly useful for the poor reader who has already ploughed through many reading books and finds that the ones which remain unread are either too difficult or of no interest. In addition, the 'language experience' approach provides an opportunity for children with poor written language skills to express themselves in writing. In the case of children with specific learning difficulties, their first language experience story may also be the first time that their thoughts have been transferred to paper. This can generate a great deal of enthusiasm.

Initially, the child composes a story orally. The story is written by the teacher exactly as the child tells it. The teacher then rereads the text to the child to see if he approves of it or wishes to revise it. This is not the time for teacher revision or criticism. The budding writer is already very reticent and it is essential to give him much encouragement in his early attempts. The story is then rewritten neatly or typewritten by the teacher. (If time allows, a typewritten version is usually preferred because it resembles a book.) The story is then used as the child's reading material but eventually the child will be encouraged to write for the other children in his class and it is suggested that authors illustrate their work.

The child's language should be preserved initially even if there are grammatical errors or incorrect usage. At a later stage it will be necessary to introduce the more formal requirements of written language as opposed to spoken language and to emphasize the greater formality of the written language register.

When compared to a phonic-based cumulative structured method, the 'language experience' approach might appear haphazard and disorganized. In fact, the stories are structured by the child's vocabulary. Children tend to repeat the same basic vocabulary and this relatively consistent repetition encourages word recognition and prediction. In any case, a phonic method can and should be used in conjunction with the language experience approach to complement it.

The beauty of the 'language experience' approach is that it is so easily predicted by its author i.e. the child. By rereading his own text, the child will recognize words which he may otherwise have never recognized, simply because he has written the text himself. In the case of spelling, the child is shown the words he will need to spell since these are the words that he is inclined to use when dictating a story. Although reading the words will almost certainly not teach him how to spell them, he will still acquire the ability to recognize them visually and this will enable him to proof-read these words at a later stage.

The main advantage of the 'language experience' approach is its role in the promotion of free writing. The initial benefits are obvious. The child is given the opportunity to produce creative writing without being in any way constrained by his limited written language ability. This new found freedom catapults a child into a world he had not previously imagined possible. In addition, the increased awareness of the communicative purpose of written language enhances motivation and interest in acquiring literacy skills.

Once the child has gained sufficient confidence in his ability to produce the thought content of free writing, he can be asked to write his own stories. Extremely poor spellers often produce stories which are virtually impossible to decipher. Usually, however, the child can remember the words he intended to use so that the teacher can correct the spelling. Sensitivity is obviously necessary. At this stage, it is desirable for the child with specific learning difficulties to learn that he has something to say. It may even be possible to fire his imagination and creative talents. Therefore, at this juncture it is important to keep the function of writing and the mechanics of writing and spelling apart so that when the child is learning to write he is not totally overwhelmed and frustrated by his inability to learn the conventions of the English spelling system.

As the child's image of himself as a good writer improves it becomes possible to apply spelling instruction to the child's stories. Instead of correcting each word the teacher may show the child words he can spell and ask him to correct them. Each story provides material for continuous assessment of spelling performance and indicates which spelling patterns the child needs to learn.

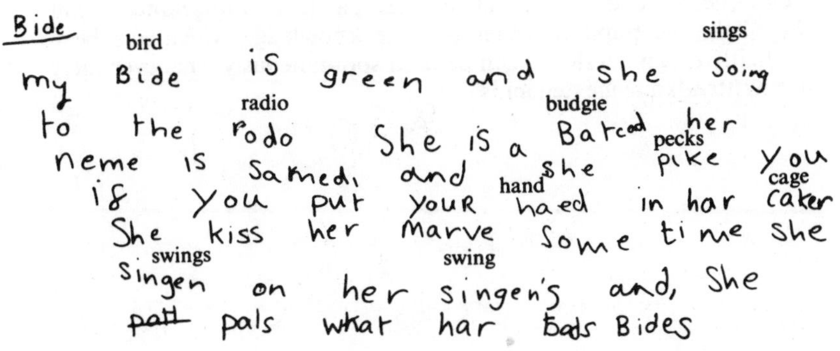

Figure 8.3 Free writing from a 12-year-old girl

This piece (see Figure 8.3), written by a 12-year-old girl, gives substantial information about her spelling ability. Phonic skills are particularly poor. See, for example, 'haed' for 'hand', 'singen' for 'swings', 'pike' for 'pecks'. She is, however, able to spell the first letter of each word correctly which indicates that simple sound–letter correspondence is available. On the other hand, she appears to remember certain words through visual memory, i.e. 'green', 'some time', 'what', and this method of remembering spellings is clearly more successful for her. She will therefore need substantial training in 'whole word' methods to reinforce her strengths and systematic phonic training to support her visual memory when it fails her.

Frequently, older children will be using words which they will not encounter for quite a while in their structured spelling programme. It is appropriate, therefore, either to introduce relevant new spelling patterns such as 'tion' so that the child can spell the words he uses most frequently or to teach them as irregular words.

Punctuation can also be taught using the child's own text. One possible technique is to add the punctuation to the text in stages. For example, the full stops and capital letters can be added first and ordered in paragraphs, then in a subsequent version commas, question marks and exclamation marks can be inserted. Finally, quotation marks can be added as well as more paragraphs, if necessary.

In the beginning, it is preferable to encourage the child to write about subjects which interest him. Gradually, as the writing improves and the child gains in confidence, the teacher can suggest topics or (in the case of the older child) introduce him to essay writing. These last steps should enable the child with specific learning difficulties to cope with the type of work which his contemporaries are producing in the classroom.

Many important supplementary teaching techniques have not been mentioned through lack of space. In practice it is preferable for teachers to devise their own games and activities and to tailor them to the ever-changing needs of their pupils. Most teachers agree that, used in combination with a structured multisensory approach, these techniques are extremely effective. Their particular importance is that they help the pupil to generalize the knowledge which has been explicitly taught so that it can be used spontaneously whenever there are written language demands.

Jean Augur

9 Guidelines for Teachers, Parents and Learners

The causes of dyslexia are as yet unknown. One thing is certain however. Dyslexia is not only a reading problem. It is a much more complicated process than simply being unable to read. The concentration on 'reading difficulties' in almost total isolation, and with complete disregard of the problems involved with writing, spelling, memory, sequencing and orientation, has led to the belief by some that dyslexia is merely a synonym for reading failure.

One of the reasons for this is that the problem may first come to light when a child starts school and is found to make little headway in learning to read and write. On the other hand, parents may have had the feeling that 'something wasn't quite right' even before the child started school, but they may have difficulty in explaining exactly what the problems are. In some cases, when they try to explain their fears to professionals they may find themselves labelled 'fussy', 'pushy' or 'over-anxious' without cause. It is very important for teachers to listen and to take careful note of the things parents say regarding their children.

Mothers in particular can be very perceptive and a great deal can be learned about the 'pre-school' child which may be useful later on. The following are extracts from two of many letters written by mothers whose fears have not been met with understanding but which say a greal deal:

'Today I am feeling cross and a bit hostile to the unfairness of others' attitudes and I know within myself I shouldn't mind so much. Tomorrow I will probably feel stronger and better and be able to cope and feel less vulnerable. Life's like that, I'm trying to understand dyslexia myself and help my son achieve what is possible for him. I don't want him hurt or his achievements belittled or undermined and I want his strengths to be acknowledged and any achievement in the things he finds difficult to be recognized for the effort he expends upon them and praised. It hurts when he asks me why I named him Jonathon and not A .... D .... a clever little boy in his class who is a good all-rounder and well advanced in the subjects Jonathon finds hard. He really believed that if we had called him another name he would be able to read! It hurt when after an eye-test he was told his eyes were beautiful and just perfect by the Doctor. He

147

said, "I know that already, it's my brain that doesn't work properly". He said it so matter-of-fact too.'

'In September last year he began school at the local primary. As soon as instruction in basic reading (flash card method) and writing began, Tim was hopelessly lost. I told his teacher and the head-mistress that I believed he was suffering from the condition known as dyslexia, since I knew from general reading that his type of speech problem was so often a sign. They refused to listen, said "it will come in time" and told me to "go home and stop worrying".

As I watched him work at home I became more convinced. Though sometimes he wrote from left to right, more often it was right to left. He persistently wrote MIT for TIM .... The most saddening aspect of all this is to see the marked deterioration in Tim's behaviour since starting school. He is basically a happy, good-natured child, but frustration, teasing etc. at school are making him bitter, bad-tempered and spiteful. This already at 6! Though his gross motor ability seems totally unimpaired, he has difficulty dressing himself, and dreads trying to put his coat on at school for fear of ridicule. Shoelaces are of course an impossibility, so he wears "heavy-duty" sandals. During his second term his teacher told me very rudely that if I had spent 10 minutes with him at home he would have no trouble with laces!'

Co-operation and liaison are necessary in all areas of education but particularly so in the field of dyslexia, about which there has been so much controversy and misunderstanding. This liaison should not be confined to a dialogue between home and school but should exist also between teachers in the same school and between schools at all educational levels, i.e. nursery, infant, junior and secondary, as the child moves on from one to the other. It is important, too, to keep open-minded. In my experience the better the teacher, the more open-minded he/she is, and the best teachers are those who find teaching a learning experience.

Much can also be learned from listening to what the children themselves say, for example:

'I think God's put my brain in upside down.'

'My brain aches.'

'My brain's gone blunt.'

'The words all get mixed up; they don't go together. You know what I mean.'

'The word's in my mouth but I can't get it out.'

'My hand didn't do what I wanted it to do.'

'Where does this book start?'

'This book is stupid. It doesn't make sense.'

'Is yesterday the day after tomorrow?'

'Is "telephone" a 3 word syllable?'

' "Xylophone" isn't in the dictionary.'

Later on some children, students and adults are able to express their anxieties in writing. The example shown in Figure 9.1 written by a 12-year-old boy points out many of the activities dyslexics find hard to do, while the final sentence expresses the despair that he is feeling.

MY LIFE AT SCHOOL

My life at school is very hard. Some teachers pick on me
or that is what I think.

The punishments I have been given are
   100 lines
   Detention
   Writing all my work out again
   Being hit over the head with a triangle and a book

Boys pick on me.

The teachers I hate are all of them except . . .

I hate my life at school. I think nobody likes me, even
my friends are horrible.

Things I find hard to do are
   Copying from the blackboard
   Doing maths

One day I had to do about 3 hours 3 minutes
homework

There is one thing they cannot take away from me and
that is my happiness.

One teacher pulled my hair for singing.

I would like to get a mighty microphone so I could tell
everyone.

There are bullies in the school trying to trip me up.

I think that everything comes apart in my hands like
when I broke the phone and smash things.

Figure 9.1 A 12-year-old boy writing about those things which he finds difficult

    The first sentences are particularly significant. It must often seem to
children that teachers 'pick on them'. This is because teachers so
frequently comment on the things which are wrong rather than on
those which are right. It is very important for teachers and parents to
set attainable targets and to develop a repertoire of 'positive responses'. Charles Cripps says in 'Catchwords': 'A negative remark
destroys a child's confidence whereas a positive comment will encourage him to communicate in writing and enjoy doing it.' It is
important to handle mistakes carefully. A mistake can be either a
stumbling block or a stepping stone to learning.

The majority of children spend most of their school day in the classroom and it is essential that this environment should be as helpful and sympathetic as possible. This chapter seeks to provide guidelines for recognizing the dyslexic child in the classroom. It also suggests ways in which parents and teachers can achieve better understanding and can cope more adequately both at home and at school.

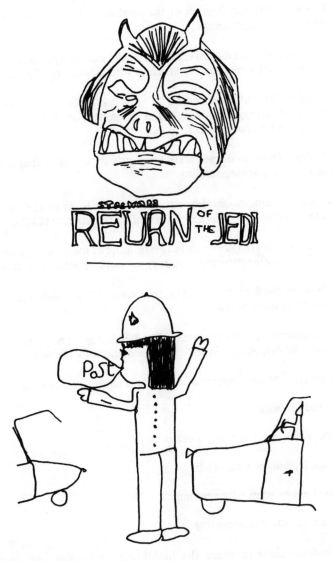

Figure 9.2 Examples of artwork from a boy aged eleven and a girl aged eight, both dyslexic

Understanding the Problem

1)   Dyslexia is not related to intelligence but it is easier to spot in a child of average or above average intelligence because of the obvious discrepancy between his intelligence level and his performance in reading, writing and spelling.

2)   There are varying degrees of the disability, from the comparatively mild to the really severe.

3)   A child of average intelligence with a mild case of dyslexia is often easier to help than a very intelligent child who is severely affected.

4)   A child of low intelligence who also displays dyslexic tendencies is in for a hard struggle although the pressures on him and the expectations of him may be less.

5)   Dyslexic children do not learn efficiently by the most frequently used methods of teaching reading.

6)   Dyslexic children who learn to read do not learn to spell at the same rate. Spelling has to be carefully and systematically taught.

7)   Dyslexic children are weak in two or more of the following areas: visual recall, visual sequencing, auditory memory, short-term memory.

8)   Dyslexic children are not lazy, careless or stupid, although they are often given these labels.

9)   The difficulty frequently runs in families and more boys than girls suffer with the disability – in my experience about five to one.

10)   Past records and reports often contain comments such as:

Could do better.

Oral work good, written work poor.

Must try harder with reading.

Must get to grips with reading.

Exam results disappointing.

11)   Dyslexic children share the inability to recognize and recall written symbols and make them into meaningful words for reading and spelling.

12) Dyslexia is not just a reading and spelling problem but affects many other areas of a child's life. Reading and spelling are the areas, however, which cause the most anxiety in a society which demands a certain degree of competence in these skills.

Early Indications

There may have been little indication before the child starts school that problems are in store. A mother who has had other children may have a 'feeling' that all is not quite well, or an enlightened doctor, health visitor or speech therapist may have expressed some concern. Once at school, however, several things soon come to light and it is at this point that an observant and caring reception class teacher can be of utmost help. The way in which she lays the foundations of his acquisition of written language could well mean the difference between success or failure in his school career. Let us look at some of these early indications.

1) Difficulty with fastening his coat, shoelaces and tie.

2) Shoes often on the wrong feet, seemingly unaware that they are uncomfortable.

3) Appears to be clumsy or 'accident prone'.

4) Difficulty hopping, skipping, or clapping a simple rhythm.

5) Difficulty throwing, catching or kicking a ball.

6) Difficulty understanding prepositions connected with direction, e.g. in/out, up/down, under/over, forwards/backwards.

7) Difficulty carrying out more than one instruction at a time.

8) Possible history of slow speech development.

9) Excessive spoonerisms, e.g. 'par car' for 'car park', 'beg and acorn' for 'egg and bacon'.

10) Difficulty in pronouncing multisyllable words, e.g. 'hopsital' for 'hospital'.

11) Difficulty in finding the *name* for an object.

12) Confusion between left and right.

13) Undetermined hand preference.

CWLD–K*

14) Poor handwriting with many reversals and badly formed letters.

15) Inability to copy accurately, particularly from the blackboard.

16) Difficulty remembering what day it is, when his birthday is, his address or his telephone number.

17) Difficulty learning to tell the time.

18) Unsure about 'yesterday' and 'tomorrow'.

19) Difficulty remembering anything in sequential order, e.g. days of the week, months of the year and multiplication tables.

20) Poor reading progress on both look–and–say and phonic methods.

21) Excessive tiredness due to the amount of concentration and effort required often for very little result.

Many of these points are still evident during the junior school years together with more specific reading and writing errors.

Reading

1) Hesitant and laboured reading especially when reading aloud, often missing out words or adding extra words.

2) Failure to recognize 'familiar' words, i.e. words that have been met and discussed many times before.

3) Misses out a line or reads the same line twice.

4) Repeatedly losing his place.

5) Confusion between similar looking words, e.g. on/no, for/of/off/from, ever/even/every.

6) Difficulty breaking down long words into syllables and putting the syllables back into the correct order. Often syllables are missed out altogether, e.g. 'frantic' for 'fantastic', 'affectedly' for 'affectionately'.

7) Disregard for punctuation.

8) Making anagrams of words, e..g 'tired' for 'tried', 'wives' for 'views', 'breaded' for 'bearded'.

9)   Difficulty picking out the most important points from a passage.

10   Inability to blend letters together.

Writing and Spelling

1)   Poor standard of written work in comparison with oral ability.

2)   Messy work with many crossings out and words tried several times, e.g. sens, cens, sns, scens, sense.

3)   Persistent confusion with letters which look alike, particularly b/d, p/g, p/q, n/u, m/w, s/z.

4)   Wrong choice of letters due to poor auditory discrimination, particularly between the short vowel sounds (ă) as in ant, (ĕ) as in egg, (ĭ) as in ink, (ŏ) as in orange, (ŭ) as in up; also between similar sounding consonant sounds, e.g. (t) and (d), (p) and (b), (m) and (n) etc.

5)   Confusion between letter *names* and *sounds* resulting in mistakes such as 'ne' for 'any', 'nd' for 'end', 'flt' for 'felt'.

6)   Indiscriminate use of capital letters usually because the child feels more secure with the capital form of the letter e.g. raBBit, muDDle.

7)   Confusion between similar sounding words, e.g. 'accept' and 'except', 'our' and 'are', 'one' and 'won'.

8)   Letters, syllables and words omitted, inserted or in the wrong order.

9)   A word spelt several different ways in one piece of writing, e.g. campping, cammping, camping, kamping.

10)   Crossing 'l' but failing to cross 't' or dot 'i', e.g. 'teller' for 'letter'.

11)   Badly set out written work.

12)   Inability to stay close to the margin.

13)   Losing the point of the story being written.

14)   Lack of or indiscriminate use of punctuation.

15)   Difficulty writing the date, e.g. 21st June 1984 (21.6.84) written as 6.12.48.

By the time a dyslexic child arrives in the secondary school, he may well be a very confused and anxious young person. With the increased amount of reading and written work expected of him, his anxiety will only increase. The discrepancy between what he should be achieving and what he is actually achieving will become more and more apparent. He may well continue to make some of the errors already mentioned. In addition, there will be others:

1)   Difficulty coping with the layout of a big secondary school. He may well lose his way and continually arrive late for lessons.

2)   Difficulty coping with a complicated timetable, particularly if it is a ten day or two week timetable.

3)   Difficulty reading aloud and a very slow reading rate when tested on a test such as the Neale Analysis of Reading Ability.

4)   Difficulty taking notes from the blackboard or from dictation which results in poor and incomplete records which in turn will be useless for revision.

5)   Examination results which do not reflect either the effort made during the term or the oral ability of the child.

6)   Poor handwriting, usually deliberately done to disguise poor spelling.

Assessment in the Classroom

If a teacher recognizes some of these examples in a child, there are several things she can do to help.

1)   Write down as much as possible about the child. Don't wait until the end of the day but keep a book and pen at the ready. The information will be invaluable.

2)   Talk to the parents. Listen to what they say, particularly if they appear to be worried. Ask if any other members of the family have experienced similar difficulties.

3)   Read all previous reports and record cards and note the comments. This includes reports from doctors, speech therapists, health visitors and social workers.

4)   Talk to his previous teachers and look at examples of his earlier written work if they are available.

5) Test the child on a non-verbal intelligence test, e.g. The Ravens Matrices or The English Picture Vocabulary Test, which will give an indication of his mental age.

6) Administer a reading and a spelling test not only to determine a reading and spelling age but how the reading and spelling ages compare with the mental age.

7) Make careful notes of the *types* of errors made in the reading and spelling tests.

8) Ask the child to do a piece of written work without asking for any help with spelling. Make a note of the time he takes over it. Use this for diagnosing the nature of the errors under specific headings:

(a) Auditory Discrimination
e.g. 'chrain' for 'train', 'pin' for 'pen'

(b) Auditory Sequencing
e.g. 'hopsital' for 'hospital'

(c) Visual Discrimination
e.g.'migth' for 'night'

(d) Visual Sequencing and Orientation
e.g. was/saw, on/no, 'paly' for 'play'

(e) Handwriting Errors

(f) Lack of Knowledge
e.g. plural rules or rules for suffix adding

9) List his reading errors under similar headings:

(a) Omissions, Additions and Transpositions of letters, syllables and words

(b) Substitutions
e.g. house/home, I/me

(d) Sequencing and Direction
e.g. out/not

(e) Lack of Knowledge
e.g. of silent 'e' or that 'c' before 'e', 'i' and 'y' sounds (s)

Reading one page from the 'Fuzz Buzz' series, a 12-year-old boy made the following errors:

a) won for now – complete reversal

b) on for no – complete reversal

c) brown for down – reversal of b/d and addition of the letter r

d) back for black – omission of second letter of initial blend

e) every for very – confusion of similar looking and similar sounding words

f) concert for contest – confusion of similar looking words

g) three for there – visual sequencing error *or* confusion of similar looking words

This boy needs sequencing and orientation exercises, auditory discriminating exercises to help him to hear the difference between single sounds and blends and 'whole word' recognition exercises, particularly of similar looking words, with emphasis on the difference between the sounds of them.

10) If parents are to be asked to help at home, clear instructions should be given on how this should be done. It is unfair to send a list of spellings home to be learned without such guidance. The same applies to reading. Parents are usually willing to help but need direction. The example, Figure 9.3, shows a page from the reading record book of a

Date	Who did you read to?	Pages	Words	Attempt	Refusals	Comments
18·11·83	Mrs. Tabona	24	flew telegraph	fell (E) telephone (E)	scene	needed help with breaking down of words with more than 2 syllables
21/11/83	Mrs Marlow	26 27	usual	usually	caution	
27/11/83	R Surmon	28 30	there crashed piled	they crashes peeled	/	worked out longer words on his own well.
28·11·83	S. M. Tibbitt	31 32	pushedpaste pulled (E)	pulled (E)		
29.11.83	A. Surmon	34 38	Crowded	rescued	slice	Read chapter well. only words as stated needed help.
	LIVING DANGEROUSLY					Well done
30/11/83	Mrs Angus	4	stood it is	Crowd (E) to (E) is (E)	worse	Good
1/12/83	R Surmon	6 & 7	GIANT THERE	GIANT THESE	/	Slow but very accurate

Figure 9.3 Page from a record book which documents a child's reading progress

child. The parents have been given instructions on how to listen to the reading, how long to continue and the way in which to fill in the record book. This is only one way of keeping an ongoing record.

The Aston Index

At the point when a teacher feels she needs further tests to confirm her diagnosis, the Aston Index may be useful. This is a classroom screening test devised to identify and assess the child with a written language difficulty. The aim is to provide a general framework for teacher observation in order to pick out the strengths and weaknesses of the child and plan an appropriate remedial programme.

The actual Index consists of two Levels. Level 1 is aimed at identifying the 'at risk' child and is administered when the child is about 5½–6-years-old after he has been in school a few months. Level 2 is aimed as a diagnostic test for older children already showing signs of failure in written language.

A word of warning – apart from the Draw–a–Man test and the Schonell spelling test, all the sub-tests must be given individually and this can be time consuming, even though they are all simple and easy to give. It is not, however, essential or necessarily desirable to administer the whole Index at one sitting.

By the time a child with difficulties is 8½-years-old, he should have been recognized, referred, assessed and diagnosed. An appropriately planned teaching programme should have begun and be well under way.

The teaching methods found to be most successful with the dyslexic child who has already started to fail are also appropriate for small children receiving their first instruction in reading, writing and spelling (see Hornsby, this volume). Prevention is better than cure and if all the children entering school were taught in a more structured manner with greater emphasis on the use of the multisensory approach, many of the children presented for remedial help would not need it. Very often children who have failed are casualties of our present teaching methods. The majority of children have a sensori-motor system which is particularly suited to the acquisition and development of both spoken and written language. In the dyslexic child, however, the sensori-motor channels, i.e. the visual, the auditory, the oral and the motor-kinaesthetic, do not appear to work in harmony, so he is unable to produce the correct automatic response to a stimulus. Multisensory learning is learning by the *simultaneous* use of eyes, ears, speech organs, fingers and muscles. The advantage of this method is that the child is able to use his areas of strength while at the same time exercising and strengthening his weaker ones. The aim is for the child to learn (for permanent automatic response) the names, sounds and shapes of all the phonograms and to develop the ability to sequence them correctly. The knowledge has to be so secure that he can produce any aspect of the symbol when needed for either reading, writing or spelling. All his perceptual systems must interact simultaneously in order for this to happen.

General Guidelines for the Classroom Teacher

1)   Let the dyslexic child sit near to you so that you can observe him and give him as much help as possible.

2)   Appreciate that he will have persistent difficulty learning anything in sequential order, especially multiplication tables. Provide him with a table chart and allow him to use it. Devise games which encourage an automatic response.

3)   Appreciate that the standard of his work will be inconsistent and erratic.

4)   However carefully he is taught anything connected with written language, e.g the silent 'e' rule, do not assume that the dyslexic child will remember and be able to use it. Constant over-learning is essential at every stage.

5)   Never indicate that he is slow, lazy or stupid or compare his written work with that of other members of the class.

6)   Do not ask him to read aloud in front of the class unless he particularly wants to do so.

7)   Judge his ability more on his oral responses than on his written answers.

8)   In the classroom generally, find other activities worthy of praise and recognition, as well as written work.

9)   Write very well and clearly on the blackboard, especially if he is expected to copy it. Check his copying or appoint someone in the class to do so. If he is copying down a homework assignment, check that he has written Page 13 Ex 6 and not Page 31 Ex 9.

10)   Be patient if he loses his way and arrives late for lessons or always appears to be in the wrong place at the wrong time.

11)   Don't expect him to use a dictionary to find out how to spell a word. Dictionaries are meant for finding out the meanings of words that you already know how to spell or for confirming or checking a spelling.

Give the dyslexic child an exercise book with a page for every letter of the alphabet. He should endeavour to open the book at the correct page for you to write in the word for him. Alternatively, have a Word Bank in the classroom where words are listed under headings. He can look under the alphabet letter or category he needs in an attempt to find the word for himself.

12)   Efficient use of the dictionary needs to be systematically and thoroughly taught. An adult dyslexic recently explained that, as she couldn't spell the word 'ridiculous', to find it in the dictionary she looked up 'silly' in Roget's Thesaurus and found 'ridiculous'!

13)   Understand that it will be necessary to provide the dyslexic child with the pre-reading type of activities for much longer than is usually considered necessary.

14)   Rhymes and poetry involving the days of the week, months of the year, the seasons and counting will be useful, also games to improve his sequential memory, e.g. 'I went to the market and I bought . . . . . .'

Reading

1)   Make sure that he is taught all the alphabet letters for name, sound and shape – upper case *A*, lower case *a* and handwritten *a*. The handwritten letter should be learnt by tracing over the top of the printed lower case letter. This technique is fully described in 'Mind your P's and Q's', which can also be used in the form of an alphabet frieze.

There should, anyway, be alphabet friezes up on classroom walls in primary school, showing all the letter formations and clue pictures for the sounds of letters. (See Figure 9.4.)

2)   Teach him which letters are the vowels and which are the consonants.

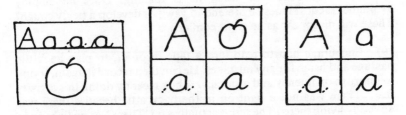

Figure 9.4 Alphabet friezes recommended for reinforcement of letter names, sounds and shapes

3)   Check that he can hear the difference between each of the short vowel sounds:

(ă) as in apple

(ĕ) as in egg

(ĭ) as in ink

(ŏ) as in orange

(ŭ) as in up

4)   Check that he can hear the difference between each of the long vowel sounds:

(ā) as in acorn

(ē) as in emu

(ī) as in ivy

(ō) as in open

(ū) as in unicorn

5)   Check that he can hear the difference between the short and long sound of the same vowel, also between similar sounding consonants, e.g. (p) and (b), (f) and (th), (m) and (n), (k) and (g) and less obvious ones, e.g. (tr) as in train, (ch) as in chain, (cr) as in cream, (kw) as in queen.

6)   Check that he knows the easier consonant digraphs, e.g. ch, sh and the easier vowel digraphs, e.g. oo, ay.

7)   Does he know the blends, e.g. st, gr, spl, and can he blend sounds together?

8)   Note his behaviour when he is reading. Does he employ avoidance tactics? Does he pretend to yawn or develop a tickly cough? These will disappear as he gains confidence.

9)   Encourage him to read into a tape recorder, to play back the passage and listen for any mistakes. He can then record it again, trying to improve on fluency and accuracy. A boy recently doing this activity read 'There was not a light on in the back attic because there was no–body living there'. The script actually said 'There was no light on in the back attic as no–one lived there'. When he listened to his recording he discovered his own mistakes.

10) Don't expect that when his reading improves his spelling will improve at the same rate – it won't. Spelling is an entirely different skill and much more difficult to acquire.

Spelling and Writing

1) Don't mark every wrong spelling – it is far too disheartening.

2) Don't give him long lists of mixed words to learn every week. Perhaps he could have fewer words or preferably a 'family' of words, e.g. fight, light, sight, might, etc. Do not include 'height' or 'straight' in this list. These are irregular and will only confuse him.

3) Copying out his corrections several times will be of little help to him. Instead, write the word out correctly for him. He should then look at it very carefully, noting any tricky parts, and write it several times over the top of the original, naming the letters as he does so. He should then cover the word and try to write it from memory. He then checks it. If it is correct he ticks it, otherwise he repeats the procedure.

4) When marking his work, don't put a line right through or under the whole of the mis-spelt word. Underline the bit of the word that is wrong or indicate where the omission or addition is. He can then have a second look and may be able to correct it himself. (See Figures 9.5 and 9.6.)

5) The dyslexic child will not notice punctuation when reading as he will be concentrating so hard on the words. It is unlikely, therefore, that he will use it in his written work and if he does, the commas are often upside-down or the full stops are 'in the air'. Careful explanation in the most precise detail will be needed.

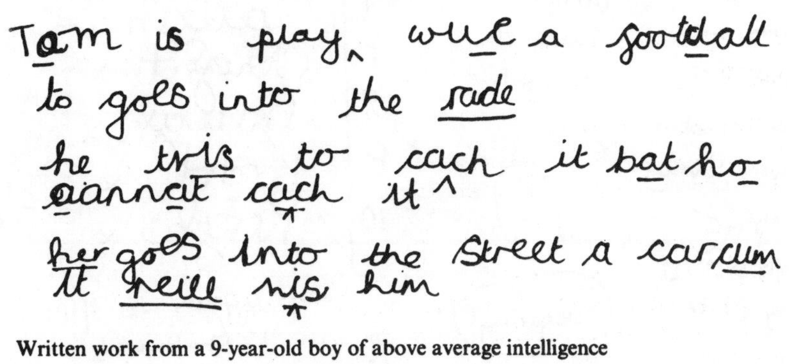

Written work from a 9-year-old boy of above average intelligence

Figure 9.5 Example of helpful marking

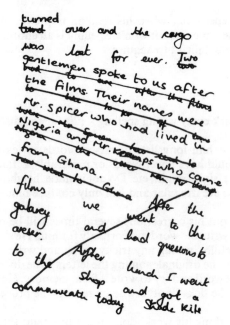

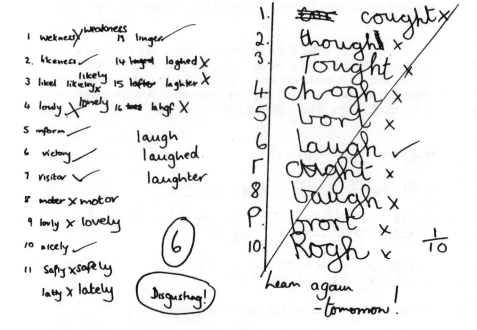

Figure 9.6 Examples of unhelpful marking

6)   Help him to order his thoughts before writing a little story (or, later, essay) so that it has a beginning, middle and end. He could tell a story on to the tape recorder first, then listen to it and perhaps write it down from the tape in his own time.

7)   He may write badly for a number of reasons – one could be to hide his poor spelling. Help him to improve his handwriting. Group similar letters together, e.g.

8)   Choose work sheets with care, making sure that they are appropriate. There is a world of difference between a *reading* exercise and a *spelling* exercise. The following is a reading exercise because the child is required to read the words, not spell them:

shop
                            The . . . is on the sea
ship

This is a spelling exercise:

c . . . . or k . . . .?
.at   .ing   .amp   .ettle

The child is required to make a spelling choice. When his answers have been checked he should study the word, write over it several times if necessary, then write it from memory.

Give him some Guidelines

1)   In every English word there must be a vowel or the letter y acting as a vowel; similarly in every syllable of every word.

2)   No English word ends with v, you must use ve.

3)   No English word ends with j – after a short vowel use dge, e.g. badge, bridge, otherwise use 'ge', e.g. cage, forge.

4)   (ij) on the end of a longer word is usually spelt –age, e.g. village, postage. There are however a few exceptions.

5)   No English words end with i, you must use y.

6)   The letter y has three sounds. Where it comes at the beginning of a word and in compound words such as 'farmyard' it is a consonant and says (y) as in yet. When it comes in the middle or the end of a word it is a vowel and has the same sound as the vowel i – that is (ī) as in lynx and (ĭ) as in fly.

7)   q is never written alone – always qu; qu never ends a word – always que.

8)   ck, ll, ff, ss, tch, dge never start English words. They always follow short vowels.

9)   c followed by e, i and y has the sound (s) as in celery, city, cyst.

10)   g followed by e, i and y has the sound (j) usually as in germ, giant, gypsy.

11)   all, full and till joined to another syllable have only one l, e.g. all + most = almost, hope + full = hopeful, un + till = until.

12)   One syllable words ending with one vowel and one consonant double the final consonant before adding a vowel suffix, e.g. clap + p + ing = clapping, scrub + b + ed = scrubbed.

13)   Vowel – consonant – e words drop the e before adding a vowel suffix, e.g. hope + ed = hoped, like + ing = liking.

14)   Words ending with a consonant and y change y to i before adding a suffix, e.g. happy + ness = happiness, beauty + ful = beautiful.

15)   Words ending with a vowel and y just add both vowel and consonant suffixes straight on, e.g. pay + ment = payment, joy + ous = joyous.

16)   The past tense suffix ed has three different sounds: (ĭd) as in patted, (d) as in filled, (t) as in jumped.

Guidelines for Parents

1)   Games such as I Spy, Snap, Pelmanism, Kim's Game and 'I went to market' are all learning games in addition to being fun. They help to improve discrimination, perception, sequencing ability and memory.

2)   Puzzle pages in comics are excellent. Joining dots, following mazes, spotting the differences, are all useful for improving hand/eye co-ordination and noticing detail.

3)   Read to children far beyond the infant school age. Tape stories for children to listen to. Look at books together, discussing pictures and diagrams. Use prepositions and words connected with direction.

4)   Watch television *together* and discuss the programmes.

5)   Encourage hobbies and special aptitudes.

6) Ask for a school timetable so that you can help to prepare the equipment needed for each day. Do not do everything for him, however, he should be encouraged to put everything ready the night before to avoid panic the following morning. A bad start is often the beginning of a bad day.

7) Take him to places of interest. If he is studying a play for 'O' Level, try to visit the theatre to see it being performed.

8) Don't allow him to make dyslexia an excuse for not working. He must work harder than others if he is to overcome his difficulty and he'll need support and encouragement every step of the way.

9) Ask the school for advice on how to hear your child read and on how best to help with spellings. Also ask for guidelines on how much help to give with homework. It is important to know the school policy regarding homework. It is inevitable that a dyslexic child will take far longer than his peers to complete an assignment. Should he continue with a 40 minute assignment until it is completed or should he stop after the 40 minutes whether it is finished or not?

10) Make use of all the 'taped' stories which are now on the market.

11) Many useful leaflets are available from the British Dyslexia Association, Church Lane, Peppard, Oxon.

Conclusions

It is important to give all children a good foundation upon which to build, but for the dyslexic it is *vital*. It could make all the difference between success and failure. The dyslexic needs structured teaching using a multisensory approach, slow and careful explanations of new concepts with consolidation for as long as necessary, and attainable targets to aim for. He needs positive reinforcement and the use of suitable worksheets, exercises, games and activities, audio-visual and computer programs.

Careful record keeping is essential and the teacher must ask herself the following questions:

1) Is this working?

2) If not, why not?

3) What do I need to do for this child?

There are no miracle cures nor short cuts, but for a hard-working child of average intelligence who is diagnosed early and is taught in a structured, cumulative and multisensory way, the prognosis is good. The final examples (Figure 9.7) show the improvement in a child's written work over a two year period using the techniques described above and advocated by the late Kathleen Hickey. The examples are taken from 'This Book Doesn't Make Sens Cens Sns Scens Sense'.

1) before tuition: an eight-and-a-half-year-old boy's attempt to write the alphabet and his name. Note the fusions.

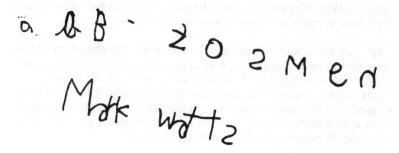

2) a few months later

... but all the tribe
had the signal
and then they
all went down to
the river and
they found a
foot print
of a tiger
and one
of the men
said, "it must be
a man eating
tiger"
So that night
all of the tribe
locked the place
up and when
the tiger
comes he ...

3) two years later: The margin at the side is for 'helpful clues'. 'Because', 'thought' and 'would' are sight words which he later worked on, using the whole word multisensory technique.

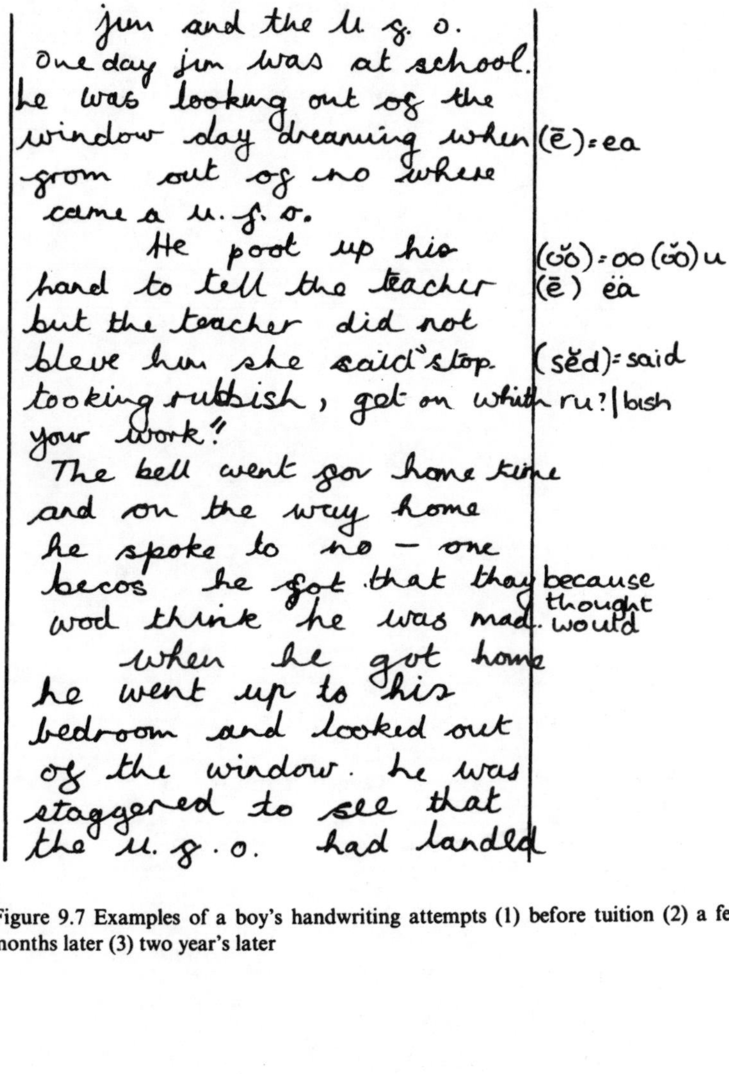

Figure 9.7 Examples of a boy's handwriting attempts (1) before tuition (2) a few months later (3) two year's later

Postscript

Margaret Snowling

Some Consistencies and Contradictions: Directions for Future Research

This book has deliberately focussed on the continuing *language* needs of children with specific learning difficulties (dyslexia). Perusal of the various contributions reveals two major themes. The first is that we are speaking of a developmental disorder, the nature of which changes through time. The second is that amongst dyslexics there are individual differences. These reflect not only constitutional differences but also the varying strategies which the children have adopted to compensate for their basic weaknesses.

The developmental perspective is introduced by Jean Cooper who draws attention to the links between early (spoken) language and later (written) language skill, and the theme is elaborated by Harry Chasty who draws our attention to changes in written language demands upon the individual. Researchers must be certain to take these points to heart; any attempt to compare dyslexic with normal readers must employ appropriate (developmental) controls.

Peter Bryant criticizes research which ignores the possibility that reading experience can affect cognitive processing. He therefore advocates the adoption of 'reading–age matched' designs in which disabled readers are compared with younger normal readers of the same reading level. Whether such a stringent match is required when children are to be compared on tasks which do not involve the presentation of written materials is arguable. For example, John Rack reviews rather convincing evidence which points to *auditory* memory deficits in dyslexia and Hanna Klein presents some striking instances of word finding difficulties in picture naming from her clinical experience. It would be wrong to dismiss these findings out of hand but, still, we need evidence that these deficits 'exist' when dyslexics are compared with controls equated for reading experience. The overwhelming prediction, judging by the pages of this book, is that the deficits will persist. It will be interesting to see if this is true and of great significance.

One area of research which has been conducted with due consideration of these points leaves us in no doubt that dyslexics have difficulty with tasks which involve phoneme segmentation. Furthermore, Joy Stackhouse shows these deficits extend into the population of children with speech disorders. However, in spite of, and indeed in considering, this evidence, Bryant makes the strong claim that dyslexics are no different from normal readers. His implicit assumption is that if dyslexics could be taught to segment better (and presumably earlier) then they would progress normally. We can say with certainty that early intervention and training in sound categorization is effective, but might there remain a hard core of dyslexics whose (phonological) deficit is such that they are not amenable to this type of training?

A more general issue is raised by the question 'Are dyslexics "different" from normal readers?' This is the issue of delay as opposed to disorder in development. Let us take as a working hypothesis that dyslexics have a phonological deficit and, therefore, their acquisition of reading and spelling is affected. If this deficit is always present to the same degree, then development can be considered to deviate from the norm. In teaching dyslexics to read and spell it would, if this were true, be prudent to foster 'alternative' strategies. The multisensory teaching approach advocated by both Jean Augur and Beve Hornsby attempts to do just this by utilizing the individual's strong senses to circumvent their weaknesses. In a similar vein, Nata Goulandris documents some of the ingenious mnemonics which dyslexics themselves devise to overcome their difficulties.

On the other hand, it could turn out that dyslexics improve their ability to use phonological codes as time proceeds. If so, we can consider their development normal, but delayed. It follows that reading and spelling would develop normally if postponed to a later date, when maturation was sufficient. But, a note of caution: reading tuition can seldom be postponed. The onus is on practitioners to ensure, perhaps by intervention, that children are ready to learn to read at the *right* time. Otherwise, a simple delay in development can rapidly escalate and look, to all intents and purposes, like a disorder.

To return to the issue of individual differences; it seems highly likely that some dyslexics will show a delayed pattern of development, whereas others will show one which deviates from normal. The appropriate research has yet to be done to tell us 'who is who'.

Thus, dyslexia is a complex condition, one which presents a puzzle to parents, a challenge to 'therapists' and a tricky set of methodological problems for researchers. Only some of the questions raised have received answers. Others will await research which considers the make-up of individual dyslexic children, how this changes with time and how it interacts with the teaching they receive.

References

Aaron, P.G., Baxter, C.F. and Lucenti, J. (1980). 'Developmental dyslexia and acquired dyslexia: two sides of the same coin?' *Brain and Language*, **11**, 1–11.

Alley, G. and Deshler, D. (1979). *Teaching the Learning Disabled Adolescent: Strategies and Methods*. Denver: Love.

Alston, J. and Taylor, J. (1984). *The Handwriting File*. Wisbech, Cambs.: Learning Development Aids.

Anthony, A., Bogle, D., Ingram, T.T.S. and McIsaac, M.W. (1971). *Edinburgh Articulation Test*. Edinburgh: Churchill Livingstone.

Atkinson, R.C. and Shiffrin, R.M. (1968). 'Human memory: a proposed system and its control processes.' In: Spence, K.W. and Spence, J.T. (Eds) *The Psychology of Learning and Motivation: Advances in Research and Theory. 2*. NewYork: Academic Press.

Aubrey, C., Eaves, J., Hicks, C. and Newton, M. (1982). *Aston Portfolio*. Wisbech: Learning Development Aids.

Augur, J. (1982). *This book Doesn't Make Sens Cens Sns Scens Sense*. Staines: Jean Augur.

Augur, J. (1983). *Mind your P's and Q's*. Staines: Jean Augur.

Baddeley, A.D. (1968). 'How does acoustic similarity influence short-term memory?' *Quarterly Journal of Experimental Psychology*, **20**, 249–64.

Baddeley, A.D. (1976). *The Psychology of Memory*. New York: Academic Press.

Baddeley, A.D. (1978). 'The trouble with levels: a reexamination of Craik–Lockhart's framework for memory research.' *Psychological Review*, **85**, 139–52.

Baddeley, A., Ellis, N., Miles, T. and Lewis, V. (1982). 'Developmental and acquired dyslexia: a comparison.' *Cognition*, **11**, 185–99.

Baron, J., Treiman, R., Wilf, J.F. and Kellman, P. (1980). 'Spelling and reading by rules.' In: Frith, U. (Ed) *Cognitive Processes in Spelling*. London: Academic Press.

Bartlett, F.C. (1932). *Remembering*. Cambridge: Cambridge University Press.

Bauer, R.H. and Emhert, J. (1984). 'Information processing in reading disabled and nondisabled readers.' *Journal of Experimental Child Psychology*, **37**, 271–81.

Beauvois, M.F. and Derouesne, J. (1979). 'Phonological alexia; three dissociations.' *Journal of Neurology, Neurosurgery and Neuropsychiatry*, **42**, 1115–24.

Benson, D.F. and Geschwind, N. (1969). 'The alexias.' In: Vinken, P.J. and Bruyn, G.W. (Eds) *Handbook of Clinical Neurology: Disorders of Speech, Perception and Symbolic Behaviour, 4*.

Berko, J. (1958). 'The child's learning of English morphology.' *Word*, **14**, 150–77.

Birch, H. and Belmont, A. (1964). 'Auditory-visual integration in normal and retarded readers.' *American Journal of Orthopsychiatry*, **34**, 852–61.

Bissex, G.L. (1980). *GNYS at Work: A Child Learns to Write and Read.* Cambridge MA: Harvard University Press.

Blalock, J. (1981). 'Persistent problems and concerns of young adults with learning disabilities.' In: Cruikshank, W. and Silver, A. (Eds) *Bridges to Tomorrow, 2.* Syracuse: University Press.

Bloom, L. and Lahey, M. (1978). *Language Development and Language Disorders.* New York: Wiley.

Boder, E. (1973). 'Developmental dyslexia: a diagnostic approach based on three atypical reading–spelling patterns.' *Developmental Medicine and Child Neurology,* 15, 663–87.

Bradley, L. (1980). *Assessing Reading Difficulties.* London: MacMillan Educational.

Bradley, L. (1981). 'The organisation of motor patterns for spelling: an effective remedial strategy for backward readers.' *Developmental Medicine and Child Neurology,* 23, 83–91.

Bradley, L. and Bryant, P. (1978). 'Difficulties in auditory organisation as a possible cause of reading backwardness.' *Nature,* 271, 746–47.

Bradley, L. and Bryant, P. (1978). 'Independence of reading and spelling in backward and normal readers.' *Developmental Medicine and Child Neurology,* 21, 504–14.

Bradley, L. and Bryant, P. (1983). 'Categorising sounds and learning to read: a causal connexion.' *Nature,* 301, 419.

Bradley, L. and Bryant, P.E. (1985). *Rhyme and Reason in Reading and Spelling.* Ann Arbor: University of Michigan Press.

Brady, S., Shankweiler, D. and Mann, V. (1983). 'Speech perception and memory coding in relation to reading ability.' *Journal of Experimental Child Psychology,* 35, 345–67.

Brainerd, C.J. and Pressley, M. (1982). *Verbal Processes in Children.* New York: Springer Verlag.

Brandt, J. and Rosen, J.J. (1980). 'Auditory–phonemic perception in dyslexia: categorised identification and discrimination of stop consonants.' *Brain and Language,* 9, 324–37.

Branwhite, A.B. (1983). 'Boosting reading skills by direct instruction.' *British Journal of Educational Psychology,* 53, 267–77.

Brimer, M.A. and Dunn Lloyd, M. (1962). *English Picture Vocabulary Test.* Bristol: Educational Evaluation Enterprises.

Bryant, P.E. (1975). 'Cross-modal development and reading.' In: Duane, D.D. and Rawson, M.B. (Eds) *Reading, Perception and Language.* Baltimore: York Press.

Bryant, P. and Bradley, L. (1980). 'Why children sometimes write words which they do not read.' In: Frith, U. (Ed) *Cognitive Processes in Spelling.* London: Academic press.

Bullock Report. Great Britain. Department of Education and Science (1975). *A Language for Life.* London: HMSO.

Butler, K. (1984). 'Adolescent language learning disorders.' *Topics in language disorders,* 4, 2.

Byrne, B. and Shea, P. (1979). 'Semantic and phonetic memory codes in beginning readers.' *Memory and Cognition,* 7, 333–38.

Campbell, R. (1983). 'Writing nonwords to dictation.' *Brain and Language*, **19**, 153–79.

Campbell, R. (in press). 'When children write nonwords to dictation.' *Journal of Experimental Child Psychology*.

Canning, B.A. and Rose, M.F. (1974). 'Clinical measurements of the speed of tongue and lip movement in British children with normal speech.' *British Journal of Disorders of Communication*, **9**, 45–50.

Carney, E. (1979). 'Inappropriate abstraction in speech assessment procedures.' *British Journal of Disorders of Communication*, **14**, 123–35.

Carver, C. (1970). *Word Recognition Test*. Buckhurst Hill, Essex: Hodder and Stoughton Educational.

Chomsky, C. (1971). 'Write first, read later.' *Childhood Education*, **47**, 296–99.

Chukovsky, K. (1963). *From Two to Five*. Berkeley and Los Angeles: University of California Press.

Cohen, R.L. and Netley, C. (1981). 'Short term memory deficits in reading disabled children in the absence of opportunity for rehearsal strategies.' *Intelligence*, **5**, 69–76.

Coltheart, M. (1980). Analysing reading disorders. Unpublished manuscript. Birkbeck College, University of London.

Coltheart, M., Masterson, J., Byng, S., Prior, M. and Riddoch, J. (1983). 'Surface dyslexia.' *Quarterly Journal of Experimental Psychology*, **35A**, 469–96.

Conrad, R. (1964). 'Acoustic confusions in immediate memory.' *British Journal of Psychology*, **55**, 75–84.

Cotterell, G.C. (1969). *Diagnosis in the Classroom*. Birmingham: School of Education.

Cotterell, G.C. (1970). 'Teaching procedures.' In: Franklin, A.W. and Naidoo, S. (Eds) *Assessment and teaching of dyslexic children*. London: I.C.A.A.

Craik, F.I.M. and Lockhart, R.S. (1972). 'Levels of processing: a framework for memory research.' *Journal of Verbal Learning and Verbal Behaviour*, **11**, 671–84.

Craik, F.I.M. & Tulving, E. (1975). 'Depth of processing and retention of words in episodic memory.' *Journal of Experimental Psychology*, **104**, 268–94.

Cronnell, B. (1978). 'Phonics for reading versus phonics for spelling.' *Reading Teacher*, December, 337–40.

Crystal, D. (1976). *'Child Language, Learning and Linguistics.'* London: Edward Arnold.

Crystal, D. (1982). *Profiling Language Disability*. London: Edward Arnold.

Denckla, M.B. and Rudel, R.G. (1976a). 'Naming of object drawings by dyslexic and other learning disabled children.' *Brain & Language*, **3**, 1–15.

Denckla, M. and Rudel, R. (1976b). 'Rapid automatised naming: dyslexia differentiated from other learning disabilities.' *Neuropsychologia*, **14**, 471–79.

Edwards, M. (1982). Verbal Dyspraxia: A Disorder of Rhythm and Seriation. Paper presented to National Conference NZST Association. Wellington, New Zealand. May.

Ellis, A.W. (1982). 'Spelling and writing (and reading and speaking).' In: Ellis, A.W. (Ed) *Normality and Pathology in Cognitive Functions.* London: Academic Press.

Ellis, A.W. (1984). *Reading, Writing and Dyslexia.* London: Lawrence Erlbaum Ass.

Ellis, N. (1981). 'Visual and name coding in dyslexic children.' *Psychological Research,* **43**, 201–18.

Fernald, G.H. (1943). *Remedial Techniques in Basic School Subjects.* New York: McGraw.

Fleming, K.J. (1971). 'Guidelines for choosing appropriate phonetic contexts for speech sound recognition and production practice.' *Journal of Speech and Hearing Disorders,* **36**, 356–67.

Fletcher, S.G. (1978). *The Fletcher Time by Count Test of Diadochokinetic Syllable Rate.* Tigard, Oregon: CC Publications Ind.

Fox, B. and Routh, D.K. (1976). 'Phonemic analysis and synthesis as word attack skills.' *Journal of Educational Psychology,* **68**, 70–4.

Francis, H. (1982). *Learning to Read: Literature Behaviour and Orthographic Knowledge.* London: Allen and Unwin.

Frith, U. (1979). 'Reading by eye and writing by ear.' In: Bouma, H., Kolers, P.A., Wrolstad, M.E. (Eds) *The Processing of Visible Language, 1.* New York: Plenum.

Frith, U. (1980). 'Unexpected spelling problems.' In: Frith, U. (Ed). *Cognitive Processes in Spelling.* London: Academic Press.

Frith, U. (1981). 'Experimental approaches to developmental dyslexia: an introduction.' *Psychological Research,* **43**, 97–109.

Frith, U. (1985). 'Beneath the surface of developmental dyslexia.' In: Marshall, J.C., Patterson, K. and Coltheart, M. (Eds) *Surface Dyslexia.* London: Routledge & Kegan-Paul.

Frith, U. and Frith, C. (1980). 'Relationships between reading and spelling.' In: Kavanagh, J.F. and Venezky, R.L. (Eds) *Orthography, Reading and Dyslexia.* Baltimore: University Park Press.

Frith, U. and Snowling, M. (1983). 'Reading for meaning and reading for sound in autistic and dyslexic children.' *British Journal of Developmental Psychology,* **1**, 329–42.

Gaddes, W.H. (1980). *Learning Disabilities and Brain Function – A Neuropsychological Approach.* New York: Springer-Verlag.

German, D.J.N. (1982). 'Word finding substitutions in children with learning disabilities.' *Language, Speech and Hearing Services in Schools,* **13**, 223–30.

Gentry, J.R. and Henderson, J.H. (1980). 'Three steps to teaching beginning readers to spell.' In: Henderson, E.H. and Beers, J.W. (Eds) *Developmental and Cognitive Aspects of Learning to Spell: A Reflection of Word Knowledge.* Newark, Delaware: International Reading Association.

Gillet, J.W. and Kita, M.J. (1980). 'Words, kids and categories.' In: Henderson, E.H. and Beers, J.W. (Eds) *Developmental and Cognitive Aspects of Learning to Spell: A Reflection of Word Knowledge.* Newark, Delaware: International Reading Association.

Gittelman, R. and Feingold, I. (1983). 'Children with reading disorders I. Efficacy of reading remediation.' *Journal of Child Psychology and Psychiatry, 24,* 167–92.

Godfrey, J.J., Syrdal-Laskey, A.K., Millay, K.K. and Knox, C.M. (1981). 'Performance of dyslexic children on speech perception tests.' *Journal of Experimental Child Psychology, 32,* 401–42.

Goldstein, D.M. (1976). 'Cognitive–linguistic functioning and learning to read in preschoolers.' *Journal of Educational Psychology, 68,* 680–88.

Goodman, K.S. (1973). 'Psycholinguistic universals in the reading process.' In: Smith, F. *Psycholinguistics and Reading.* New York: Holt, Rhinehart and Winston.

Grunwell, P. (1980). 'Developmental language disorders at the phonological level.' In: Jones, M. *Language Disability in Children.* Lancaster: MTP Press.

Grunwell, P. (in press). *Phonological Assessment of Child Speech (PACS).* Windsor: NFER-NELSON.

Hickey, K. (1977). *Dyslexia – A Language Training Course for Teachers and Learners.* Kathleen Hickey Publications.

Hornsby, B. and Shear, F. (1976). *Alpha to Omega.* London: Heinemann Educational Books.

Howell, J. and Dean, E. (1983). 'Phonological disorders revisited.' *Bulletin of the College of Speech Therapists, 377,* 11–13.

Hughes, R. (1983). 'The internal representation of word–final phonemes in phonologically disordered children.' *British Journal of Disorders of Communication, 18,* 79–89.

Hulme, C. (1981). *Reading Retardation and Multisensory Learning.* London: Routledge and Kegan Paul.

Ingram, T.T.S., Mason, A.W. and Blackburn, I. (1970). 'A retrospective study of 82 children with reading disability.' *Developmental Medicine and Child Neurology, 12,* 271–81.

Ingram, D. (1981). *Procedures for the Phonological Analysis of Children's Language.* Baltimore: University Park Press.

Johnson, D.J. (1980). 'Persistent auditory disorders in young dyslexic adults.' *Bulletin of the Orton Society, 30,* 268–76.

Johnson, D.J. and Myklebust, H. (1967). *Learning Disabilities: Educational Principles and Practices.* New York: Grune and Stratton.

Jorm, A.F. (1979). 'The cognitive and neurological basis of developmental dyslexia: a theoretical framework and review.' *Cognition, 7,* 19–33.

Jorm, A.F. (1983), 'Specific reading retardation and working memory: a review.' *British Journal of Psychology, 74,* 311–42.

Kellet, B., Mobley, P. and Lee, B. (1984). *Kellet Colour Coding Programme.* Manchester: Central Manchester Health Authority.

Kirk, S., McCarthy, J. and Kirk, W. (1968). *The Illinois Test of Psycholinguistic Abilities*. Urbane: University of Illinois Press.

Kirk, U. (1983). *Neuropsychology of Language, Reading and Spelling*. New York: Academic Press.

Klapp, S.T., Marshburn, E.A. and Lester, P.T. (1983). 'Short term memory does not involve the 'working memory' of information processing: the demise of a common assumption.' *Journal of Experimental Psychology*, 112, 240–64.

Klatzky, R.L. (1975). *Human Memory: Structures and Processes*. San Francisco: Freeman.

Lea, J. (1970). *The Colour Pattern Scheme: A Method of Remedial Language Teaching*. Oxted, Surrey: Moorhouse School.

Lerner, J. (1981). *Children with Learning Disabilities*. Boston: Houghton and Mifflin.

Levinson, P.J. and Sloan, C. (1980). *Auditory Processing and Language: Research and Perspectives*. New York: Grune and Stratton.

Lewkowicz, N.K. (1980), 'Phonemic awareness training: what to teach and how to teach it.' *Journal of Educational Psychology*, 72, 686–700.

Liberman, I.Y. and Shankweiler, D. (1979). 'Speech, the alphabet and teaching to read.' In: Resnick, L. and Weaver, P. (Eds) *Theory and Practice of Early Reading*. Hillsdale, N.J.: Lawrence Erlbaum Associates.

Liberman, I.Y., Shankweiler, D., Liberman, A., Fowler, C. and Fischer, F.W. (1977). 'Phonetic segmentation and recoding in the beginning reader.' In: Reber, A.S. and Scarborough, D.L. (Eds) *Towards a Psychology of Reading*. Lawrence Erlbaum Associates.

Lucas, E.V. (1980). *Semantic and Pragmatic Language Disorders: Assessment and Management*. London: Aspen Systems.

Lundberg, I., Olofsson, A. and Wall, S. (1981). 'Reading and spelling skills in the first school years predicted from phonemic awareness skills in kindergarten.' *Scandinavian Journal of Psychology*, 21, 159–73.

Luria, A.R. (1966). *Higher Cortical Functions in Man*. London: Tavistock.

Marcel, T. (1980). 'Phonological awareness and phonological representation: investigation of a specific spelling problem.' In: Frith, U. (Ed) *Cognitive Processes in Spelling*. London: Academic Press.

Marsh, G., Friedman, M., Welch, V. and Desberg, P. (1980). 'The development of strategies in spelling.' In: Frith, U. (Ed) *Cognitive Processes in Spelling*. London: Academic Press.

Menyuk, P. (1963). 'Syntactic structures in the language of children.' *Child Development*, 34, 409–630.

Menyuk, P. (1969). *Sentences Children Use*. Cambridge MA: M.I.T. Press.

Menyuk, P. and Bernholtz, N. (1969). 'Prosodic features and children's language production.' *Research Laboratory of Electronics: Quarterly Progress Reports*, 93.

Miles, T. (1974). *Understanding Dyslexia*. London: Priory Press.

Miles, T.R. (1982). *Dyslexia: The Pattern of Difficulties*. London: Granada.

Montgomery, D. (1981). 'Do dyslexics have difficulty accessing articulatory information?' *Psychological Research*, 43, 235–43.

Morrison, F.J. and Manis, F.R. (1982). 'Cognitive processes in reading disability: a critique and proposal.' In: Brainerd, C.J. and Pressley, M. (Eds) *Progress in Cognitive Development Research*. New York: Springer-Verlag.

Myklebust, H.R. (1983). *Progress in Learning Disabilities, 5*. New York: Academic Press.

Naidoo, S. (1972). *Specific Dyslexia*. London: Pitman Publishing.

Neale, M.D. (1958). *Neale Analysis of Reading Ability*. Southampton: MacMillan Educational.

Nelson, D.L. and Borden, R.C. (1978). 'Encoding and retrieval effects of dual sensory–semantic cues.' *Memory and Cognition, 5*, 457–61.

Nelson, H.E. and Warrington, E.K. (1974). 'Developmental spelling retardation and its relation to other cognitive abilities.' *British Journal of Psychology, 65*, 265–74.

Nelson, H.E. and Warrington, E.K. (1980). 'An investigation of memory functions in dyslexic children.' *British Journal of Psychology, 71*, 487–503.

Newton, M. and Thomson, M.E. (1976). *The Aston Index*. Wisbech, Cambs.: Learning Development Aids.

Olofsson, A. and Lundberg, I. (in press). 'Can phonemic awareness be trained in kindergarten? '*Scandinavian Journal of Psychology*.

Perfetti, C.A. and Hogaboam, T. (1975). 'The relationship between simple word decoding and reading comprehension skill.' *Journal of Educational Psychology, 67*, 461–69.

Perin, D. (1983). 'Phonemic segmentation and spelling.' *British Journal of Psychology, 74*, 129–44.

Personke, C. and Yee, A.H. (1971). *Comprehensive Spelling Instruction: Theory, Research and Application*. Scranton, Pennsylvania: International Textbook Company.

Peters, M.L. (1967). *Spelling: Caught or Taught?* London: Routledge and Kegan Paul.

Peters, M.L. (1970). *Success in Spelling: A Study of the Factors Affecting Improvement in Spelling in the Junior School*. Cambridge: Cambridge Institute of Education.

Peters, M.L. and Cripps, C. (1978). *Catchwords: Ideas for Teaching Spelling*. London: Harcourt Brace, Jovanovich.

Phelps-Gunn, T. and Phelps-Terasaki, D. (1982) *Written Language Instruction: Theory and Remediation*. London: Aspen.

Piaget, J. and Inhelder, B. (1973). *Memory and Intelligence*. London: Routledge and Kegan Paul.

Pollock, J. (1978). *Signposts to Spelling*. London: Helen Arkell Centre.

Posner, M. (1969). 'Abstraction and the process of recognition.' In: Spence, J.T. and Bower, G. (Ed) *The Psychology of Learning and Motivation, 3*. London: Academic Press.

Rack, J. (in press). 'Orthographic and phonetic encoding in normal and dyslexic readers.' *British Journal of Psychology*.

Rak, E. (1977). *Spellbound*. Cambridge MA: Educators Publishing Inc.

Rak, E. (1977). *The Spell of Words*. Cambridge MA: Educators Publishing Inc.

Read, C. (1971). 'Preschool children's knowledge of English phonology.' *Harvard Educational Review*, **41**, 1–34.

Read, C. (1975). 'Lessons to be learned from the preschool orthographer.' In: Lennenberg, E.H. and Lennenberg, E. (Eds) *Foundations of Language Development, 2*. London: Academic Press.

Robertson, S. (1984). Children's strategies in the development of reading and spelling. Unpublished D.Phil Thesis; University of Oxford.

Robinson, P., Beresford, R. and Dodd, B. (1982). 'Spelling errors made by phonologically disordered children.' *Spelling Progress Bulletin*, **22**, 19–20.

Rodgers, B. (1983). 'The identification and prevalence of specific reading retardation.' *British Journal of Educational Psychology*, **53**, 369–73.

Rozin, P. and Gleitman, L. (1977). 'The structure and acquisition of reading II: the reading process and the acquisition of the alphabetic principle.' In: Reber, A.S. and Scarborough, D.L. (Eds) *Towards a Psychology of Reading*. Hillsdale, NJ: Lawrence Erlbaum Associates.

Rugel, R.P. (1974). 'WISC subtest scores of disabled readers.' *Journal of Learning Disabilities*, **7**, 48–55.

Rutter, M. and Yule, W. (1973). Specific reading retardation. In: Mann, L. and Sabatino, D. (Eds) *The First Review of Special Education*. Philadelphia: Buttonwood Farms.

Rutter, M. and Yule, W. (1975). 'The concept of specific reading retardation.' *Journal of Child Psychology and Psychiatry*, **16**, 181–97.

Schonell, F.J. (1942). *Backwardness in the Basic Subjects*. Edinburgh: Oliver and Boyd.

Seymour, P.H.K. and McGregor, C.J. (1984). 'Developmental dyslexia: a cognitive experimental analysis of phonological, morphemic and visual impairments.' *Cognitive Neuropsychology*, **1**, 43–82.

Shallice, T. (1981). 'Phonological agraphia and the lexical route in writing.' *Brain*, **104**, 413–29.

Shankweiler, D., Liberman, I.Y., Mark, L.S., Fowler, C.A and Fischer, F.W. (1979). 'The speech code and learning to read.' *Journal of Experimental Psychology: Human Learning and Memory*, **5**, 531–45.

Shear, F., Raines, J. and Targett, D. (1977). *Space to Spell*. Bath: Better Books.

Shear, F., Raines, J. and Targett, D. (1977). *More Space to Spell*. Bath: Better Books.

Slobin, D. (1971). *Psycholinguistics*. Glenview, Illinois: Scott Foresman.

Snowling, M.J. (1980). 'The development of grapheme–phoneme correspondence in normal and dyslexic readers.' *Journal of Experimental Child Psychology*, **29**, 294–305.

Snowling, M.J. (1981). 'Phonemic deficits in developmental dyslexia. '*Psychological Research*, **43**, 219–34.

Snowling, M.J. (1982). 'The spelling of nasal clusters by dyslexic and normal children.' *Spelling Progress Bulletin*, **22**, 13–18.

Snowling, M.J. and Perin, D. (1983). 'The development of phoneme segmentation skill in young children.' In: Rogers, D.A. and Sloboda, J.A. (Eds) *Acquisition of Symbolic Skills.* New York: Plenum Press.

Snowling, M.J. and Stackhouse, J. (1983). 'Spelling performance of children with developmental verbal dyspraxia.' *Developmental Medicine and Child Neurology*, 25, 430–37.

Spring, C. and Capps, C. (1976). 'Encoding speed, rehearsal and probed recall of dyslexic boys. '*Journal of Educational Psychology*, 66, 780–86.

Stackhouse, J. (1982). 'An investigation of reading and spelling performance in speech disordered children.' *British Journal of Disorders of Communication*, 17, 53–60.

Stackhouse, J. (1984). 'Phonological therapy: a case and some thoughts.' *Bulletin of the College of Speech Therapists*, 381, 10–11.

Stackhouse, J. and Snowling, M. (1983). 'Segmentation and spelling in children with speech disorders.' In: Edwards, M. (Ed) *Proceedings of XIX Congress of the International Association of Logopaedics and Phoniatrics.* Edinburgh: College of Speech Therapists.

Stagg, D. (1984). *PSM 1.* Cheltenham: Stanley Thornes Publishers Ltd.

Stanovich, K.E. (1980). 'Toward an interactive-compensatory model of individual differences in the development of reading fluency.' *Reading Research Quarterly*, 16, 32–71.

Sweeney, J.E. and Rourke, B.P. (1978). 'Neuropsychological significance of phonetically accurate and phonetically inaccurate spelling errors in younger and older retarded spellers.' *Brain and Language*, 6, 212–25.

Tansley, P. and Panckhurst, J. (1983). *Children with Specific Learning Disabilites.* Windsor: NFER-NELSON.

Temple, C. and Marshall, J.C. (1983). 'A case study of developmental phonological dyslexia. '*British Journal of Psychology*, 74, 517–33.

Thomson, M.E. (1982). Reading and spelling errors in dyslexic children: delayed or deviant? Paper presented to BPS Cognitive Psychology Section Conference on Dyslexia. Manchester.

Thomson, M.E. (1982). 'Assessing the intelligence of dyslexic children.' *Bulletin of the British Psychological Society*, 35, 94–6.

Torgeson, J. and Goldman, T. (1977). 'Verbal rehearsal and short term memory in reading disabled children.' *Child Development*, 48, 56–60.

Valett, R. (1980). *Dyslexia: A Neuropsychological Approach.* London: Aspen.

Van Kleek, A. (1981). 'Children's development of metalinguistic skills: implications for assessment and intervention with language disordered children.' *Communicative Disorders*, 6.

Vellutino, F.R. (1977). 'Alternative conceptualization of dyslexia: evidence in support of a verbal deficit hypothesis.' *Harvard Educational Review*, 47, 334–54.

Vellutino, F.R. (1979). *Dyslexia: Theory and Research.* Cambridge. MA: M.I.T. Press

Vellutino, F.R. Pruzek, R, Steger, J.A. and Meshoulam, U. (1973). 'Immediate visual recall in poor readers as a function of orthographic–linguistic familiarity.' *Cortex*, 9, 368–84.

Vogel, S.A. (1974). 'Syntactic abilities in normal and dyslexic children.' *Journal of Learning Disabilities*, **7**, 103–09.

Wallach, G.P. and Butler, K.G. (1984). *Language Learning Disabilities in School-Age Children*, London: Williams and Wilkins.

Winer, F. (1970). *Phonological Process Analysis*. Baltimore: University Park Press.

Winer, F. (1981). 'Treatment of phonological disability using the method of meaningful minimal contrast: two case studies.' *Journal of Speech and Hearing Disorders*, **46**, 97–103.

Wendon, L. (1978). *The Pictogram System*. Cambridge: Pictogram Supplies.

Wepman, J.M. (1958). *Auditory Discrimination Test*. Chicago: University of Chicago Press.

Wiig, E.H. and Becker-Caplan, L. (1984). 'Linguistic retrieval strategies and word finding difficulties among children with learning disabilities. *Topics in Learning Disorders*, **4**, 3.

Wiig, E.H. and Semel, E.M. (1976). *Language Disabilities in Children and Adolescents*. Columbus OH: Charles E. Merrill.

Wiig, E.H. and Semel, E.M. (1980). *Language Assessment and Intervention for the Learning Disabled*. Columbus OH: Charles E. Merrill.

Wiig, E.H. Semel, E.M. and Crouse, M.B. (1973). 'The use of English morphology by high risk and learning disabled children.' *Journal of Learning Disabilities*, **67**, 457–65.

Williams, J. (1980). 'Teaching decoding with an emphasis on phoneme analysis and phoneme blending.' *Journal of Educational Psychology*, **72**, 1–15.

Wilson, B. and Moffat, N. (1984). *Clinical Management of Memory Problems*. London: Croom Helm.

Wren, C.T. (1983). *Language Learning Disabilities: Diagnosis and Remediation*. London: Aspen Publications.

Young, J.Z. (1978). *Programs of the Brain*. Oxford: University Press.

Yule, W. (1967). 'Predicting Reading Ages on Neale's Analysis of Reading Ability.' *British Journal of Educational Psychology*, **37**, 252–55.

Yule, W., Lansdown, R. and Urbanowicz, M.A. (1982). 'Predicting educational attainment from WISC-R in a primary school sample.' *British Journal of Clinical Psychology*, **21**, 43–6.

Yule, W., Rutter, M., Berger, M. and Thompson, J. (1974). 'Over and under achievement in reading: distribution in the general population.' *British Journal of Educational Psychology*, **44**, 1–11.

Index

acquired dyslexia 53
adult dyslexia 25–26
'Alpha to Omega' 120
articulation 110
  difficulties 71
assessment
  classroom 156–157
  of learning difficulties 60, 80, 101
  of reading strategies 86
Aston Index 85, 102, 106, 158
auditory
  discrimination 102
  memory 103
  organization 103
  skills 102

case history 61
case studies 53, 60, 62, 65, 66, 75, 88,
  106, 127–132
classroom guidelines 160
cleft palate 96
coding 30–31, 32, 39
communication 12–13
compensation 41–42
comprehension 87, 106
control groups 29, 51–53
conversation 72
creative writing 69, 145–146

deficits 28–42, 52, 71
development 23–25, 29, 42, 173
  of reading and spelling 81–82, 135
dictionary work 142
dyslexia 11–15, 21, 26, 28, 44, 147–154,
  174
  dyseidetic 88–89
  dysphonetic 88–90
  phonological 54–55, 99
  surface 54–55
dyspraxia, verbal 96

Edith Norrie Letter Case 111, 143–144
elaboration 40
epidemiological studies 50
essay writing 145–146

Fernald technique 137
free writing 145

games 142–143, 166

handwriting 122, 155

intervention 115
I.Q. 44

language 15, 17–19, 59
  disability 59–78
  experience approach 144–146
  needs 44, 59–78
learning
  disability 3–7, 59
  to read and spell 82
letter–sound rules 54, 121–125, 136–137,
  165
linguistic
  concepts 68
  skills 64–78

management 59, 109
memory 34–41, 72, 72–78, 92–103
methodology 28–29, 51–53, 173
mnemonics 37, 139–140
models
  of reading 19, 98
  of spelling 90, 100
multiplication tables 75
multisensory 64, 75, 113–114, 119, 125,
  135–136, 159

naming 30–32, 62, 69
nonword reading 54
number skills 23

orthography 40, 82, 84

parents 61, 151–167
phoneme
  awareness 52–53, 81
  –grapheme skills 109
  segmentation 32–34, 91, 96–109, 112
phonological 39–40, 81, 89
  disability 97
  dyslexia 54–55, 99
prediction 44–56
predictive studies 44–50
preschool child 14–15, 42, 45–46, 82,
  104, 153
prevention of learning difficulties 43
production of spoken language 69–73
proof-reading 141

reading 80, 106, 134
  and spelling rules 114, 121
  comprehension 87, 106
  errors 88, 106, 157
  in dyslexia 47–49, 52, 154
rehearsal 37–39
remediation 161
rhyme 40, 46, 56, 113
  detection 103, 113

production 103–104, 113

school-age child 20, 153, 158
segmentation 83, 173–174
sentence structure 125
sequencing 73, 83
short-term memory 16, 35
Simultaneous Oral Spelling 138
sound categorization 112
specific learning difficulties 3–7, 11–12, 96
specific reading retardation 44, 51
speech 96, 101–107
   perception 33
   production 34, 36
   therapist 3–7, 59, 101, 109–115
spelling 21–22, 48–49, 80, 96–109, 134, 155
   difficulty 84
   errors 91, 107, 129, 132, 145–146
   models 90, 100
   remediation 46–49, 56, 163
   strategies 90–94
standardized tests 84, 106–107

story telling 72
strategies awareness 108
surface dyslexia 54–55
syllable segmentation 105, 112
syntax 65

teachers 151
teaching 49, 128, 134–146
treatment 120

understanding spoken language 62–69

verbal
   coding 32, 39
   deficit hypothesis 30
   deficits 28–42, 52, 71
   dyspraxia 96
visual
   coding 30–32
   strategies 87
vocabulary 62–67

whole word learning 137
writing remediation 165